C000182192

100 things
to do while
Breastfeeding

Melissa Addey

Published by Letterpress Publishing
Cover and Formatting: Streetlight Graphics

Epub: 978-0-9931817-2-6
Smashwords: 978-0-9931817-3-3
Kindle: 978-0-9931817-0-2
Paperback: 978-0-9931817-1-9

Dedicated to Seth and Isabelle: for their
joint 1500 hours and counting!
and to Ryan: for everything

Contents

700 Hours And Counting: Why I Wrote This Book

L ET'S SAY YOU FEED YOUR baby every three hours. That's about average. So you are feeding eight times in twenty-four hours. I'm going to err on the very conservative side here and say that each feed lasts half an hour. I can hear many of you snorting already. I know my daughter took at least an hour to feed for her first few weeks and I have many friends for whom an hour was a mere trifle, their babies stretching out feeding sessions into what appeared to be whole days. But bear with me. I'm trying not to exaggerate in any way. So we have eight feeds lasting half an hour each – so that's four hours every day. Times seven days a week is twenty-eight hours. Times four weeks to make a month, and let's say for the sake of argument that you feed your baby for six months, though plenty of people continue breastfeeding for much longer than that. You're now looking at close to *seven hundred hours* spent breastfeeding, and as I said, I'm erring heavily on the conservative side. You could well be clocking up double or even triple that.

If there's one thing you don't have enough of, as a parent, it's time. So losing seven hundred hours over six months (that's about two waking months of your life, by the way) to a process where you sit still and stare into space seems like a waste. Yes, of course you can gaze lovingly at your baby (see the number one suggestion in this book) but I'm not sure that doing that for seven hundred hours is really a good use of your time – or that you will fail to bond with your baby if you take your eyes off them for some of that time.

Sometimes it is bliss to just sit still and do nothing at all while your baby feeds, especially if you have a lot on or several children. I suggest you enjoy those moments! But sometimes it would be nice to be doing something for yourself as well as for your baby. Some of the suggestions here are a one-off, some could become a habit. Some may sound odd, some may sound dull. Some may not be relevant to you, for example if you don't have older children then the section on that will be of little interest (for now). But with one hundred ideas, I am sure there's something in here for you. If you invent some more things to do, let me know and I'll share them with other mothers! melissa@melissaaddey.com

I think you will find breastfeeding more rewarding, more interesting and more fun if you are enjoying yourself. I hope that somewhere in this book you will find some suggestions that suit you and your life.

Welcome to *100 things to do while Breastfeeding.*

Some assumptions...

OF COURSE YOU CAN BREASTFEED anywhere, so for all I know you spend all your breastfeeding sessions climbing the Eiffel Tower, on a train across the Australian outback, out dancing in a club and doing your yoga class. If so then I take my hat off to you. But if you've chosen to look at this book then I'm going to make some assumptions. I'm assuming that a fair few of your breastfeeding sessions are actually at home sitting down and that this book will be helpful to you for those moments where you feel a little bored and aren't sure what else you could be doing whilst breastfeeding. I'm also assuming you'll use it when you get a chance to *decide* what you'd like to be doing (as opposed to feeding whilst eating/cleaning/doing a million and one other things). So most but not all of my suggestions are for when you are at home, sitting down and with the option to choose what you'd like to do. You'll probably be on maternity leave, but there are also suggestions relevant to when you're back at work. I'm also assuming that at these moments you'll be mostly one-handed. If you are bottle-feeding there are plenty of suggestions here that can work for you too, but perhaps not all of the one hundred as you'll be holding a bottle with what would usually be your spare hand, hence my emphasis on breastfeeding. There is also a way of breastfeeding called biological nurturing (see resources at the back of the book) which allows the baby to find the breast by itself and may leave you with two hands free, in which case, many suggestions will be easier!

I'm also assuming that you and your baby are pretty comfortable with breastfeeding. I know some people may struggle at first: do ask for help and find out what works best for you. Once you've got the hang of it then you'll be relaxed and ready to try out some of these ideas without worrying about how the feeding itself is going. A few tips if you're new to breastfeeding:

learn some different positions to feed in so that you can find the best ones for you (La Leche League and the NCT can both help with this) and create a few 'nesting' spots round the house where you can comfortably feed. Keep a little basket at each spot with water, muslins, nipple cream, pen and paper, books and other useful devices you can bring along to each like a smartphone, which is an invaluable tool as a new mum with only one hand and a lot to do! If it takes you an extra twenty seconds to get set up so you are comfy and happy, I suggest your baby can wait that long even if they are fussing for their food. Better they fuss a tiny bit longer than you get stuck for possibly an hour, uncomfortable and bored. I think your baby will feed better if you are happy and relaxed.

Bond with your baby

I KNOW IT'S A COMPLETE CLICHÉ, but that's because it's true: your baby will grow up faster than you can ever imagine. My baby daughter held her head up today and wanted to be sitting up, not lying down and I suddenly saw that a part of her babyhood had already gone, even though she is still only a few months old. Even on your busy days and when you are tired, occasionally take a moment to relish each stage of your baby's changing life. So this first section is all about bonding with your baby. Since you are already holding your baby and feeding them, you are of course already bonding, but in this section I list a few extra things you can do to make this intimate time even more special for you and your baby. If you can add some of these activities to your usual breastfeeding sessions even once a day you will create a lovely special time that you will look back at with fondness. You will be helping your baby to form its deep attachment to you and you to your child.

1

Gaze at your baby

You won't need me telling you to do this at the beginning, you'll be too in awe of the tiny new life you have created not to gaze at them all the time, let alone when you're breastfeeding. But when some time has passed and you are tired, busy and have a million other things to think of, take a moment again to look down at the beautiful special person you are holding and be happy. They will get bigger and wriggle away from you when you try to hug them for more than a few seconds and you will miss this soft togetherness. Marvel at every part of them and meet their eye, then smile. As they get bigger they will break off feeding to give you a gummy smile back, which is very sweet. Often my babies made me laugh by peering up at me while feeding, one eye kept open to check up on me and make sure I was still who they thought I was. As they got older they wanted to see what I was up to while they were feeding: my five-month old son started batting his hand behind him trying to stop me focusing on my Kindle, keen that I spend all my time looking only at him. Enjoy gazing at your baby.

'Tis love that makes the world go round, my baby.

Charles Dickens

2

Massage your baby

M Y FIRST BABY GOT A full massage every day, complete with warm bath and oils. My poor daughter, coming second to a much busier mother, got the odd belly rub if she looked like she had bellyache and occasionally a fully clothed massage when I had a few minutes to spare. But if you're breastfeeding and have one spare hand, you can massage your baby. Their head, back, one arm and leg will probably all be accessible to you on each side. You can go to a baby massage class or get a book to refine your technique but even gentle rubbing and stroking will be pleasant to them and easy for you. If it's warm weather or you have a nice warm room, remove some clothing so they have skin-to-skin contact with you, which is beneficial to small babies' wellbeing – and yours. Some babies may be more sensitive to touch than others and find it distracting, but see if they can get used to the sensation over time in small doses. Massage can help a baby's digestion and studies have shown that babies who are massaged sleep better – and we all want babies who sleep better!

When you massage someone, the levels of oxytocin go up in the brain, and oxytocin is one of the chemicals that drives attachment.

Helen Fisher

3

Sing to your baby

YOU DON'T NEED TO BE able to sing in tune: lullabies, pop songs and half-remembered snatches of tunes from adverts are all good. Or make up a tune and the words as you go along – your baby will not know the difference. You can sing about what a lovely baby you have or how you are feeling. Your baby will enjoy the sound of your voice and it's a way of sharing happy memories, annoying tunes that won't get out of your head and childhood favourites with your little one. My son very kindly sang Baa Baa Black Sheep for his baby sister the first time he saw her, one of my fondest moments of them together, so rope in your other children if they are around to help you out. Singing makes you feel good too, as it releases endorphins (feel good chemicals) and will make you breathe deeper if you sing good and loud! You may create rituals and special memories through singing. My friend invented *The Cheese Song,* which was simply a litany of many, many kinds of cheeses, running to thirty-plus verses. I have a song I only sing to my children if they are ill, while a colleague at work told me they regularly played a particular song to their baby when she was tiny, only for her to unknowingly choose it to be played as she arrived for her wedding, thirty years later. It's hard to feel down if you're singing so give it a go on your 'off' days and see if it cheers you up. And who knows, you may be raising a musical child thanks to your off-key renditions of ancient chart hits.

Melissa Addey

Every heart sings a song, incomplete, until another heart whispers back. Those who wish to sing always find a song. At the touch of a lover, everyone becomes a poet.

Plato

4

Talk to your baby

I F YOU REALLY CAN'T BRING yourself to sing (or the neighbours have started complaining) then just talk. Tell your baby all about your long list of things to do, tell them how much you love them, tell them what a pain work is being, tell them what you fancy for lunch. Ask them questions and make up silly or realistic answers. As with singing, your baby will enjoy hearing your voice and you can let out frustrations, re-order your mind, pass on happy thoughts and get up from breastfeeding feeling ready for the next part of your day. Try not to be too negative (no one, not even babies, likes hearing someone be endlessly down) but let out things that are troubling you quickly and let them go, then move on to happier things. This miniature 'talking cure' might well make you feel more positive and as babies are very attuned to feelings they may benefit from your improved emotional state. Whisper nonsense too. I sometimes sat and murmured all the ridiculous pet names we had for each baby, which made me giggle and feel closer to the sleepy little bundle I was holding.

Melissa Addey

The most influential of all educational factors is the conversation in a child's home.

William Temple

5

Clip your baby's fingernails

CUTTING BABY FINGERNAILS IS ONE of the worst jobs going. Their hands are so tiny and they either keep them clenched or flail them about, neither of which helps you access the tips of their fingers. People suggest nibbling their nails off (I never dared) or using teeny-tiny clippers, which I did but still managed on a couple of occasions to clip their skin rather than their nails, which makes you feel like the very worst mother in the world as they turn puce with rage and pain and scream the place down for a few moments. Still, it has to be done, so while breastfeeding is often a good time. They are otherwise engaged, have a hand spare right next to you and are relaxed enough not to move too much. You will need some help, perhaps from your partner or a friend or even an older child if they can hold the baby's hand steady for you, but use this time to creep up on them and clip their nails before they get so long they start scratching their own face and yours. You'll find that grooming your baby is quite a nice way to bond with them (once it's all over).

Love begins by taking care of the closest ones – the ones at home.

Mother Teresa

6

Read up on the baby stuff

A USEFUL THING TO DO WHILE breastfeeding is to read up on various baby books/forums etc. for information you need or want. I had a good book called *Your Baby Week by Week* (Dr Caroline Fertleman and Simone Cave), so each week one breastfeeding session was given over to reading up on what the next week would be bringing so that I felt ahead of the game (ha!). If you're a fan of a particular baby 'guru' and their routines then you can remind yourself of the finer details of their suggestions and if you're on baby number two or more, you can be reading up on why this one is totally different from your first and how to adapt to them. You can look up ailments, how-tos and developmental milestones, as well as activities and games to do with your baby once they've finished feeding. It's also a good time to remind yourself of vaccination timetables, local baby activities and so on. In the early days of your first baby especially this is a good activity as you can read up on how to give them a bath, how to look after their cord stump and so on. And of course, the most interesting subject of all: how to get your baby to sleep – longer, better or just at all. You'll finish your feed feeling like you know a whole lot more about your baby than you did when you started and better able to care for them.

The more that you read, the more things you will know. The more that you learn, the more places you'll go.

Dr. Seuss

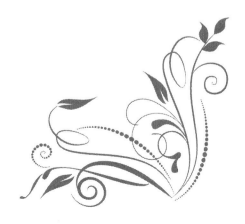

7

Write a letter to your baby for the future

Yes, your writing may be cramped and untidy but give it a go anyway. Write a letter to your baby for the future. Tell them how you feel right now, their birth story, how it felt bringing them home, their siblings' reactions, how they look and feel and sound, what you think their character is like right now. Talk to them about their surroundings and the things you think will happen in their childhood. Talk about how much you love them and your hopes, fears and dreams for their future. It doesn't matter if it's not written on scented vellum, write it on a scrappy piece of a notepad and put it away for them to read when they are older. It will be a cherished piece of writing and doing this activity will make you feel closer to your child. It can also be cathartic, if for example you had trouble conceiving or carrying a child, to acknowledge their safe arrival and your feelings along the way. Again, babies are sensitive to feelings, so if you think this will be a very upsetting exercise, it might be best to do it at another time, but if the overall feeling is positive then this is a lovely activity to do while holding your baby in your arms.

Sending a handwritten letter is becoming such an anomaly. It's disappearing. My mom is the only one who still writes me letters. And there's something visceral about opening a letter – I see her on the page. I see her in her handwriting.

Steve Carell

8

Practice mindfulness

THIS IS A SIMPLE BUT very powerful exercise: simply be mindful of the moment you are in. Focus on everything your senses can offer you: the feel of your baby sucking on your breast, the smell of their hair, the feel and weight of them in your arms, the softness of their skin and so on. Yes, you'll be breastfeeding for 700 or more hours, which seems like a lot now, but you'll be surprised how quickly this time will come to an end. Enjoy the moment and the sensation of breastfeeding for what it is and you will remember it long after it is gone with fondness and a strong physical memory.

With mindfulness, you can establish yourself in the present in order to touch the wonders of life that are available in that moment.

Nhat Hanh

Feel good: mind, body and soul

T HE EASIEST THING TO DO, as a parent, is to have your own self and needs swept away by the demands and needs of your children. You love them and so you want to put them first, but in actual fact this may not always be such a good idea. Yes, they matter, but so do you, their mother, and it is a good thing to make sure that your own needs and desires don't disappear altogether. With this in mind, this section focuses on looking after your own wellbeing: mind, body and soul. You really can't look after someone else well when you are worn out on all these levels. You will be a better mother if you are happy, nourished and strong in yourself.

9

Eat

WITHOUT FAIL, EVERY TIME I sat down to eat a meal, my baby would wake up and cry, just as the fork touched my lips. Both my children did this and it was maddening. So plan around your baby and make sure you, too, get fed. Set up a snack tray with healthy filling food that you can eat while you breastfeed, so that if you get short-changed at the table you can make up for it later. Try not to let it all be biscuits and chocolates: breastfeeding supposedly helps you lose your baby weight, but it's not a miracle worker. Oat biscuits, nuts, fruit or carrots, little packs of healthy cereals that can be eaten dry and so on can all be left out of the fridge and snacked on when you need them. Ideally, of course, someone could bring you a nice hot plate of food while you breastfeed but this may not always be possible. But do make sure that you are getting the food you need – after all, you need to keep up your energy levels and you have to produce food for another human. Try also not to get too hungry before you eat, as that's when it's easy to make poor food choices.

A crust eaten in peace is better than a banquet partaken in anxiety.

Aesop

10

Drink

NOT A G AND T, although it is tempting! It's good to stay hydrated – for your general health but especially when having to produce milk. Your body knows this and you will no doubt feel horribly thirsty every time you breastfeed. So make sure you have bottles of water on standby in your key breastfeeding spots. I found refillable bottles with sports caps on good for drinking one-handed without knocking them over by mistake in the middle of the night. Water is a great first port of call but other drinks can be good to make sure you get some nutrition in you (see eating, earlier). There are special breastfeeding teas to encourage milk production and herbal teas to help with various ailments from feeling gassy (common after a caesarean for example – peppermint tea is ideal) to helping you relax and sleep (camomile). Pure fruit juice (not 'juice drink' which will contain added sugar and water) can count towards your five a day but bear in mind it is high in natural sugars and more than one glass does not count. Milk can be good for a calcium boost. Being well hydrated will make you feel better physically and mentally, so drink up!

Water is the driving force of all nature.

Leonardo da Vinci

11

Sleep

A<small>H SLEEP, THE DESPERATE QUEST</small> of every new parent and especially the poor woman who has to repeatedly feed a crying baby in the middle of the night! All is not lost however. Once you have really got to grips with breastfeeding, try feeding your baby while lying on your side with them lying next to you. It may take some practice (perhaps start when you are quite awake!), but eventually you may well be able to sleep while feeding the baby, or at least doze. Even a little extra sleep is always a bonus, so do try this option out. La Leche League and the NCT can offer more advice on safe co-sleeping. With care, this position can give you just a little more sleep, and every little helps.

Sleep is the best meditation.

Dalai Lama

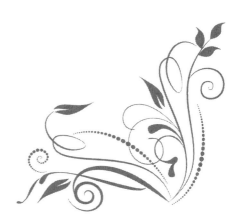

12

Smooth out your feet

I LOVE TO WALK AROUND BAREFOOT, so my feet tend to get very hard on the balls and the heels, which doesn't really look very elegant in sandals. For this activity you need one of those small handheld pedicure gadgets, essentially they have a small rotating bit of sandpaper (I know, I'm making it sound very sophisticated), which you use to get rid of the rough bits on your heels and the rest of your feet. They are not too expensive and work very well, though the replacement heads are a bit pricey. Still, it's a good present to ask for if friends or family would like to pamper you. Sit on the bed to breastfeed, pop a used towel under your feet (the dead skin will fall onto it like a powder – ewww!) and smooth one foot at a time with whichever hand you have free as the feed progresses. It can be quite satisfying to finish a feed with nice smooth feet – and then next time you could set up a footspa to finish off your tootsies nicely! The gadgets are not very noisy so they shouldn't disturb your baby. Alternatively, pop a foot mask on your feet and rest them on a towel for the duration of the feed. Roughly wipe it off/in when you're done and relish your new smooth feet.

Melissa Addey

Keep your eyes on the stars, and your feet on the ground.

Theodore Roosevelt

13

Read the Sunday papers

R EADING THE SUNDAY PAPERS MAY seem like a thing of
the past – lounging in bed of a Sunday morning with only
your partner beside you after a long and lazy lie-in. But they don't
have to be gone forever. Get your favourite one/s delivered, then
if necessary spend the rest of the week slowly working your way
through them in small chunks and get back that feeling of leisure,
albeit in small doses. Little glimpses of your former life are always
quite comforting when you're getting used to parenting for the
first time and besides, all too soon your kids will be teenagers and
you'll have read all the Sunday papers before they even wake up in
the mornings. The Sunday papers are also usually a good source of
ideas for new recipes, new outings, new books to read and so on,
so you may get some good suggestions for more things to do while
breastfeeding – or for when you have both hands free! This can also
be a nice way to spend precious time with your partner discussing
things you are reading as you go along which are not just baby-
related (see later section on staying in love with your partner).

Read a lot – poems, prose, stories, newspapers, anything. Read books and poems that you think you will like and some that you think might not be for you. You might be surprised.

Michael Morpurgo

14

Meditate

D ON'T HAVE TIME FOR YOUR meditation class or even for an
at-home session all to yourself? Try and meditate during a
breastfeeding session – even just a brief session can be a calming
and centring activity. If you are new to meditation but would
like to give it a try, if only to escape the mayhem around you and
the chaos in your brain, then just sit quietly and breathe. Notice
your breath go in and out of you and let everything else go. If
thoughts come up (as they will, of course: about what to make
for dinner, about where you put your watch, about whether you
remembered to do something) then just notice them and set them
aside for later. You may feel silly at first or that you are not doing
it 'right', but there is no right or wrong with this exercise, it is
just a moment of stillness in your life – and we could all do with
a few more of those. If you get interrupted, don't worry. Try again
at the next available opportunity. You may find that this activity
becomes a welcome and regular part of your routine and that you
may even continue it when you are done with the breastfeeding.

Half an hour's meditation each day is essential, except when you are busy. Then a full hour is needed.

Saint Francis de Sales

15

Make your hair shine

IF YOU ARE REALLY QUITE super-organised and your baby's patterns are well known to you then you might be able to set up a hair-dyeing opportunity while you breastfeed. Easier, though, would be to use a hair mask or simply leave your usual conditioner in for much longer than you usually do (a minute or so is not really enough for most of them to do the work they are intended for). Wash or wet your hair, slather on the product you have chosen, stick one of those ever-so-elegant plastic shower caps on and a towel over the top (the warmth should help the product penetrate better and you won't get a cold head) and settle down for the breastfeeding session. Afterwards, rinse it out and enjoy your lovely soft and shiny hair. Another good hair care idea is to put some olive oil or coconut oil on dry hair, rub it in, leave for a while and then wash it back out. Don't put too much on or your shampoo will struggle to get it all out again, but it does do wonders for your hair condition. And of course, the other hair care activity you can do is settle down with a hair magazine and choose your next style.

Forget not that the earth delights to feel
your bare feet and the winds long to play
with your hair.

Khalil Gibran

16

Get some fresh air

IF YOU ARE LUCKY ENOUGH to have a garden or even a terrace, then take your baby out there for a spot of feeding. Alternatively, visit your local park. Unless it's very chilly, so long as you are both well dressed you will not be too cold. If you've been feeling cooped up then this activity can really lift your spirits. On a pleasant day it can be lovely to have the breeze caress your skin, feel the sun on your face (or even work on your tan), enjoy the smell of the flowers around you and perhaps watch your other children playing. On a hot day, dabble your toes in a paddling pool and have a refreshing drink to hand. You can also plan your garden tasks while sitting outside and looking about you. Do watch out for your baby's delicate skin though: use good sun protection or stick to the shade. Another alternative is to sit on the front doorstep and watch the world go by. I did this while on maternity leave with my first baby when my husband was due home and it became a ritual of 'waiting for Daddy' that continued with my second baby. It's a great way to meet or get to know the neighbours as well, who will chat to you as they pass, which can be nice if you are feeling a bit isolated. If you don't have some outdoor space available then sit by the window with your best view, open it up, put a vase of flowers or a houseplant near you and pretend!

Beauty surrounds us, but usually we need
to be walking in a garden to know it.

Rumi

17

Keep up with the activities you love

I LOVE TO GO TO DANCE classes, it's the only kind of exercise I've ever enjoyed. Sadly having kids sort of cut down on the time I had available to do this, but watching dance shows on TV did make me feel like I was learning new steps while enjoying the music and costumes. Don't lose track of what you love: even if you can only keep up with it on TV for a while, like watching favourite sports; or playing the piano one-handed (there is actually sheet music for this!) then go for it. I think it's important that having children does not mean you have to drop everything else in your life, especially the things that you love to do and which make you the person you are. So think of the things you really miss doing and find a way to introduce them back into your life – if you're missing art then at the very least get a wonderful art book, print or calendar and put it where you can see it often. At best – go to an art gallery, find a good place to sit and do your breastfeeding there! And so on. Whatever you love to do, find a miniature way to reintroduce it into your life so that when the time is right you can build it back in again, full-size.

If you do what you love, it is the best way
to relax.

Christian Louboutin

18

Set up a footspa

I F YOU HAVE A FANCY footspa that you've never quite got round to using, now is its time. Fill it up, switch it on and you're away. If not, a simple bucket or basin filled with warm water with the addition of perhaps some Epsom salts or a few drops of essential oils that you enjoy will do the trick just as well. Do check which essential oils you shouldn't use while breastfeeding if you have a wide range to pick from or have had reactions to them in the past, but lavender, citrus or ylang ylang should all be fine. This can be a very relaxing experience and will help to revitalise your tired feet after a day spent rushing about. Some people suggest using a few spoonfuls of powdered milk and almond oil for a milk bath to rival Cleopatra's. This is a good activity to do if you're breastfeeding on your bed: start by sitting on the edge of the bed to feed. Have a towel or bath mat ready on the bed for when you finish, in case you are still feeding. Once you've had enough, lift your feet out of the water onto the towel and rotate your feet in circles, first one way and then the other. By the time you're done with the breastfeeding and stand up again, you'll have a newly refreshed pair of feet ready to go!

Be sure you put your feet in the right place, then stand firm.

Abraham Lincoln.

19

Pop your pills

I F YOU'RE SAT THERE WITH a bottle of water by your side (see the earlier point on being well hydrated) then you might want to add some pills to your next sip. Research what vitamins or supplements might be good for you and have them handy so you don't forget to take them. It's easy to put everyone else first when you have children or indeed to forget to look after yourself at all when there's a new baby in town but even a little extra care of yourself will make a big difference to your health and how you feel on a daily basis. For example, 70% of adults in the UK are lacking in Vitamin D, which contributes to the proper absorption of calcium, amongst other minerals. Read up on what supplements might be useful for your own needs and keep them where you won't forget to take them. If you don't like taking supplements then think about what vitamins and minerals you might be in need of and see what you can eat to get them naturally, for example you could snack on a little handful of nuts to help grow stronger hair and nails.

There's a world of difference between feeling OK and feeling fabulous.

Dr Wendy Denning

20

Read the online
forums for support

O NE OF THE BEST EMAILS I ever read was from one of the NCT mums I know. The subject header just said *aaarrgghh!,* which immediately made me feel better because she was having as crap a day as I was. If you're having a bad day or your child is doing something maddening/exhausting/incomprehensible/ worrying then chances are so is someone else's – and chances are it's normal. So without believing *everything* you read, do turn to the online forums now and then. I've used Mumsnet, NCT and La Leche League but you will no doubt find ones that suit you. This is how I found out that your breast milk can turn salty (which is why my baby would only drink from one breast till I pumped out the salty milk – no midwife I've ever spoken to knew about this but I believed it once I tasted it and later it happened to a friend too – pass it on!), that everyone else's toddler seemed to be waking at 5am too and that yes, your first child's regression starts *before* the new baby arrives. Many forums will have apps so you can use them easily on your phone and some sites will send you weekly or daily updates relating to the age of your baby, which you can read while breastfeeding. It's good to know you're in the same boat as other people and that the virtual community is there for you, even at 2am. My husband now regularly asks, "What do the forums say?" in the hopes that someone, somewhere, will have solved our latest parenting issue.

Melissa Addey

People are very reluctant to talk about their private lives but then you go to the Internet and they're much more open.

Paulo Coelho

21

Listen to music

MUSIC CAN CHANGE YOUR MOOD quite radically. It can cheer you up, it can calm you down and it can give you back your energy on an exhausting day. I suggest you make up a playlist of your favourite music – or even multiple ones for different mood shifts as required. Your favourite piece of music can usually make you smile, so know what it is and have it to hand so you can change the day's tempo. If you're feeling like there's nothing in your life but baby stuff then ask for new music as a gift or tune in to a radio station that suits your tastes – or even try something entirely new. I happen to be very bad at keeping up with new singers and musicians but my sister often sends me new music that makes me feel like I am not so out of touch after all.

Music is a moral law. It gives soul to the universe, wings to the mind, flight to the imagination, and charm and gaiety to life and to everything.

Plato

22

Watch the sky go by

WHEN WE GOT A LOFT conversion in our house we also got a velux window and suddenly it was like having a moving picture frame of the sky – clouds drifting by, birds flying past, the stars at night. If you have a window where you can see the stars, enjoy them during the night feeds by leaving your curtains a little bit open. In the daytimes enjoy the shapes of clouds and the wind rushing through trees – and if your baby has seen fit to want feeding as dawn breaks, at least enjoy the sunrise. We very rarely take the time to watch such things because we are too busy, but here you are with time to look out of a window and see how the world changes without us even noticing. Looking out of the windows is how I know that we are on the flight path of a local heron who fishes in one park to our east and one to our west and flies over our house between shifts.

Look up at the stars and not down at your feet. Try to make sense of what you see, and wonder about what makes the universe exist. Be curious.

Stephen Hawking

23

Watch comedy

THE FIRST TIME I SAW stand-up comedian Billy Connolly on a video I was unwell, lying on the sofa and wanted something to cheer me up. I laughed so hard I had to actually stop the video so that I could get my breath back. Don't just watch any old thing on TV: watch some comedy. Old classic sketch shows, new stand-up comedians, TV panel shows, funny films or your favourite sitcom re-runs, it's all good. Also, now is the time to watch any comedian who talks about having children. You will previously not have understood why other people were laughing *quite* so hard – but now you will because whatever was happening to them is happening to you. Even clichéd routines about how hard it is to leave the house quickly/without the kitchen sink once you have children will now become gaspingly funny to you and you'll end up with tears in your eyes, mostly because it's true rather than funny. If you're having a down day, make an effort to find something funny to watch and feel the difference it makes to your mood. Comedy shows have been fixing arguments between my husband and I for years: by the time you've laughed together at something for half an hour you've forgotten or forgiven what you were rowing about.

A day without laughter is a day wasted.

Charlie Chaplin

24

Play games

WHEN ALL ELSE FAILS AND you have a phone or a game player to hand, play something stupid to shut out the world. *Solitaire, Candy Crush, Angry Birds... Call of Duty* (!), whatever. It doesn't matter. What matters is that you will forget whatever it was you were having to deal with and just deal with very small insignificant things like a pack of cards, tiny sweeties or furious avians. You can of course (given a handy partner) also play things like board games together, which can be fun. If you want to go all Grand Master about it you can also play things like chess and Scrabble with people online, since you can do one move at a time and come back the next time you're feeding. You can rediscover old favourites from your childhood or try out the latest game everyone's been going on about. This idea does not, however, work quite as well if you are inclined to get in a rage because you can't manage to knock things down satisfactorily, shoot up enough zombies or your winning score is not your personal best. If that's the case, perhaps you'd be better off with the meditation suggestion I made earlier. You can also of course grab a pack of cards and play solitaire, which can be quite meditative. Alternatively, start studying the rules of bridge, poker and other card games and challenge your friends next time you're all together. Maybe Las Vegas won't know what's hit it!

Each player must accept the cards life deals him or her: but once they are in hand, he or she alone must decide how to play the cards in order to win the game.

Voltaire

25

Pray

YOU MIGHT HAVE A PARTICULAR faith, in which case reading your holy book, reflecting on spiritual matters or praying may all be positive and uplifting things for you to do and ones with which you are familiar and find comforting. Some people read one page a day of a spiritual text, for example, or have a time when they take a moment to say a prayer. If you are not religiously inclined, you may still have an interest in matters spiritual and in this case you can develop your own spiritual progress or rituals and undertake them while breastfeeding. You could even take this time to understand a little about other people's faiths and by doing so understand others better. Prayers do not need to be religious in nature if this is not for you, they can be simple expressions of hopes and fears, reflections and dreams. Try making a prayer you are happy with, whatever your beliefs, and say it or think it from time to time. Try it once even if you think this suggestion is not for you. You may surprise yourself.

Prayer is not asking. It is a longing of the soul. It is daily admission of one's weakness. It is better in prayer to have a heart without words than words without a heart.

Mahatma Gandhi

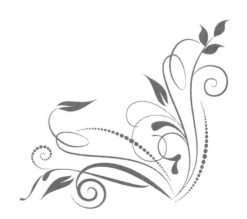

26

Moisturise

IF YOU'RE LIKE ME THEN when you get kids you'll find you are suddenly washing or wiping your hands a lot more, because you're changing nappies, doing a lot of laundry, mopping up all kinds of unmentionable things, dealing with a lot of bodily fluids and assisting with other people's toiletry needs. Ewww. And the net result of this is that your hands get very dry. Your feet and other parts of you may also end up dry because let's face it there's a lot less 'pamper time' for yourself. But here's a good idea. If you know a feed is about to take place then grab a pot of moisturiser – whatever your favourite is – and slap it on: feet, one hand, elbow, whatever's accessible. Slather it on pretty thickly and don't worry about doing a tidy job of it. Then feed your baby. By the time you've finished, it'll have sunk in and you can wipe off whatever hasn't leaving you feeling considerably smoother. My feet went from what genuinely felt like crocodile skin to something approaching human as a result of a couple of sessions of this. Yes you can use high-end products but frankly anything moisturising will do: what most products require to work at their best is the quantity and time to sink in and as we rarely have that time you don't always get the full benefit, just like hair conditioner. So smooth on the moisturiser and feel the scales turn back to skin.

I love to put on lotion. Sometimes I'll watch TV and go into a lotion trance for an hour. I try to find brands that don't taste bad in case anyone wants to taste me.

Angelina Jolie

27

List your blessings

THERE WILL INEVITABLY BE A day where life with children isn't quite what you'd hoped for: too much crying, not enough sleep, too many nappies to change, not enough milk for a sudden growth spurt leaving you with a baby attached to you like a limpet for hours. Take a deep breath and start listing the good things in your life. Start with the fundamental stuff: having enough to eat and drink, a roof over your head and take it from there. List tiny things (your electric toothbrush is freshly recharged and there's still loo roll left in the cupboard) if that's all you can think of. You might even make yourself giggle and that's a good thing. If you can find big happy things such as a loving family and great friends, a good partner (even if they are annoying you right now this minute) and your health then keep going until you've listed them all. Go back into your past, look into your future and get as many good things as possible listed in your head (or even on a piece of paper if you need hard evidence). Feel your spirits lift as you focus on the good in your life. When you are feeling better, think of one thing that will improve whatever made you feel down in the first place. Just one. Don't get caught up in listing bad things or you'll be back at square one. Just find one small action – giving your partner a hug or putting the dishwasher on – that will improve the current situation. As soon as you've finished breastfeeding, go and do it. Feel blessed in the life you have and make it better one tiny step at a time.

What if you gave someone a gift, and they neglected to thank you for it – would you be likely to give them another? Life is the same way. In order to attract more of the blessings that life has to offer, you must truly appreciate what you already have.

Ralph Marston

28

Pluck your eyebrows

I DO GENERALLY THINK THAT SUGGESTING a mother will feel great just because she's got a coat of nail polish on when what she really wants to do is get a new job, paint a great work of art or deal with serious family problems is trite and superficial beyond words, not to mention patronising. However, sometimes it is easy to make sure that the house is clean, emails have been replied to and your children are clean, fed and amused whilst you haven't even had a chance to have a shower and get dressed. This happens to me from time to time and in these instances just having hot water on me, a bit of face cream and wearing proper clothes makes me feel like I matter too. If what makes you feel like you have been looked after is to pluck your eyebrows, apply lipstick or mascara, brush your hair or put on your earrings then I say make everyone wait while you do that. You deserve to have a moment to yourself and if small actions of pampering are what make you feel human then make time for them. Yes they are superficial and yes I am sure you have bigger, better and more important things to do in your life, but your feelings matter too and if you're feeling sub-human then I doubt the other stuff will get a look in. So identify what it is that makes you feel like you can knock the world into shape and go and do it now.

Melissa Addey

A woman whose smile is open and whose expression is glad has a kind of beauty no matter what she wears.

Anne Roiphe

29

Exercise

I KNOW! LET'S DO A FULL aerobic workout whilst breastfeeding!
I'm kidding. I am the least exercise-prone person you will ever
meet. But I feel bad that I'm doing nothing and there *are* things
you can do whilst breastfeeding. If you're a truly fitness-focused
person then have a look at your usual routine and see what can
be managed. I tried out a few things just to see if they were
physically possible and I can tell you that you could actually do
things like leg lifts and bicep curls with weights while feeding
your baby, if you were so inclined. I'm not, as it happens. But
I have been known to rotate my neck and ankles, flex my feet
back and forth and do a few stretches of different limbs – oh,
and the all-important pelvic floor exercises. It's not much but it's
something, especially if you're getting over a caesarean as I was.
You can also sit cross-legged or on the ground with your legs out
to the sides to get a little bit of stretching going on. Just try one
or two things. Feeling good about that may lead to you making
a little bit of time to exercise when you're not feeding: I finally
got round to doing some stomach crunches which were much
needed. If nothing else, wriggling your shoulders may release
some stress when you've had a hard day.

It is a shame for a man to grow old without seeing the beauty and strength of which his body is capable.

Socrates

30

Exercise your face

I F THE BICEP CURLS SOUND awful, then try out something simpler and less tiring: facial fitness. You can find face yoga, face fitness and face workouts to follow from DVDs to books and apps for your phone. Because you're toning up the muscles that support your facial skin, using these exercises is supposed to keep your face away from the need to Botox or similar: and really, it would be better to look like yourself (on a great day) rather than someone else... The exercises are fairly simple, for example 'the giraffe', which involves stretching your neck up really high (head tilted back a bit) and lightly stroking your neck skin downwards. Easy! Look up a few exercises and try out the ones you can do while breastfeeding. You never know, it might take away the effect of all the sleepless nights... or at least improve matters a little. Your baby won't care if you make a few weird faces, they may even find it as entertaining as mine did: she broke off to laugh at me and then carried on feeding, content with having an oddball for a mother.

Keep your face to the sunshine and you cannot see a shadow.

Helen Keller

31

Cherish your body

Take a moment to think about the parts of your body you love the most, from your nicely shaped earlobes to your perfect feet. Then think about the parts of your body that you don't view with such enthusiasm and try to find good things about them. For starters, your stretch marks are the result of your body having created a baby, an extraordinary feat and one you can justly be proud of. Take every part of your body, from your hair down to your toenails and either see the beauty or find some, whatever it takes and however convoluted your reasoning. You'll be surprised at how positive an exercise this is. As an example, the women in my family are, ahem, *blessed* with marvellously sturdy ankles, but to be fair we are not known for twisting them either, which my husband, with his far more elegant specimens, does quite frequently. So maybe there is a positive reason for their solidity, despite their lack of superficial charm. Find the good and the beauty in your own body and be grateful for it.

Melissa Addey

There is more wisdom in your body than in your deepest philosophy.

Friedrich Nietzsche

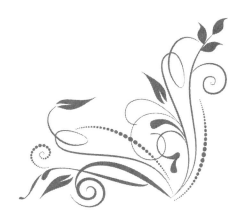

32

Dry skin brushing

Dry skin brushing is good for your circulation and supposedly improves cellulite, as well as getting rid of old dry skin. Get a long-handled brush with natural fibre bristles and gently brush your skin towards your heart. Okay, you'll probably only be able to manage your legs while breastfeeding but it's a good start. Ideal if you can time this just before a shower. My own legs get very dry and flaky so this does wonders for them. See if you can manage this: dry skin brush during one feed, then fit in a shower (ha!) and then at your next feed apply moisturiser in industrial quantities and let it soak in. Super-legs here we come!

What spirit is so empty and blind, that it cannot recognize the fact that the foot is more noble than the shoe, and skin more beautiful than the garment with which it is clothed?

Michelangelo

33

De-fuzz your legs

I KNOW YOU'RE THINKING THIS IS a bit boring but sometimes it's good to get the dull stuff out of the way leaving you time to do something more interesting for yourself later with the free time. You'll probably need an electric razor or an epilator for this but once you're settled in a good position then you can easily do one leg at a time while breastfeeding and be done and dusted and ready to do something more fun once you've finished feeding the baby. Give it a try: certainly my legs got zero attention for about two months after my babies were born so I could have done with figuring this out earlier. Top tip though if you're new to an epilator: you might want to try it out a few times without breastfeeding as the first few times are likely to be the most painful and you might not want to frighten your baby with yelps of pain!

Darling, the legs aren't so beautiful, I just
know what to do with them.

Marlene Dietrich

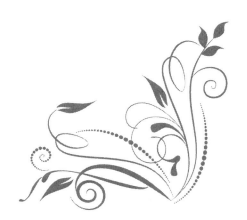

34

Put on a face mask

You may frighten the baby of course, but if you quickly put on a face mask before you start breastfeeding then by the time you've finished you'll have given your face a nice treat while feeding your little one. Drop me a line, by the way, if you manage to do multiple things while breastfeeding: face mask, footspa, eating a snack and reading a book all at the same time? You're a marvel, ma'am. You can buy ready-made masks, make your own (e.g. mashed up avocado, honey and oatmeal) or if time is limited then just use your usual face cream but slather it on in large quantities and let it sink in for a bit longer than usual. Just like your usual hair conditioner I'm betting you don't usually use enough or leave it on for long enough so this is its chance to work properly. You'll probably have to wipe down your eyebrows afterwards if you don't want to look decidedly odd but it's a small price to pay for your skin getting a much-needed 'drink'.

Man is least himself when he talks in his own person. Give him a mask, and he will tell you the truth.

Oscar Wilde

35

Whiten your teeth

No, I'm not suggesting a mobile dentist should visit you in your home, but you can do a couple of things to get whiter teeth if yours are getting neglected. My teeth were lucky to get brushed once a day in the first few weeks of juggling two children. One is to take your toothbrush with you while you breastfeed and brush for the proper full two minutes that are recommended, especially if you have an electric toothbrush. If your teeth get one extra decent clean a day for a few weeks I think you'll see some benefits. Second, of course, you can use one of those tooth-whitening kits. I will say I tried one once and didn't like the temporary extra sensitivity that I got afterwards, however that may not be the case for you. If it's something you always meant to try but never got round to sitting still long enough for, then now's your chance. And if neither of those two works for you then simply apply some really red lipstick and watch your teeth grow magically white in seconds.

She laughs at everything you say. Why?
Because she has fine teeth.

Benjamin Franklin

36

Watch films

M ANY CINEMAS HAVE MOTHER AND baby screenings, where a bit of crying won't bother anyone and you can catch up on the latest releases. If your local cinema doesn't offer this, suggest it to them or just go along to a screening at a quiet time of day (the certificate of the film will need to be suitable, e.g. a U or PG) and see how you get on. You can always leave if your baby gets upset and is bothering other people. My first baby was excellent at this activity: he would feed and then sleep throughout films, so if you miss going to the cinema for the big screen experience then do try this out. It made me feel like I was a real grown-up again after a couple of months of staying at home with a little baby and missing one of my favourite activities. If the big screen isn't an option then use this time to catch up on films you've missed in the past or even sign up to one of the many internet-based film subscriptions available to see films pretty quickly after they are released. See some old classics, catch up on your favourite film stars' careers or go all out and create themed seasons to get through.

When people ask me if I went to film school I tell them, 'no, I went to films.'

Quentin Tarantino

37

Paint your nails

I F NON-CHIPPED NAIL POLISH IS the thing that makes you feel like you are on top of the world, then use the time while breastfeeding to get someone to do this for you (even I am not suggesting you can paint your own nails while breastfeeding!). If you're brave, ask your older children but I'm telling you right now that I will not be held responsible for the result. If you're lucky enough to have a friend visiting, get them to do it. And if you want a real pampering experience, then get a mobile beautician to visit you and do a proper job. Do keep the room well ventilated though, as nail polish fumes aren't the best for anyone to breathe in. There are some more natural versions around which you could look into. You could also club together with a bunch of local mums and have a breastfeeding/nail polishing session together if you fancy making it a social occasion and the price is likely to be more affordable.

Actually, I wear the nail polish to hide how grubby my nails are.

Caroline Corr

38

Call in a mobile hairdresser

M Y MOTHER IN LAW HAS a mobile hairdresser who comes to her and does her haircut and colouring and a friend's at the same time, turning her living room into their own personal salon. If your baby isn't ready to be left at home or going to a salon with one in tow isn't your idea of relaxation, then see if there's a mobile stylist who can come to you. They might even be able to do your older children's hair while they're at it (and your partner's?), making their visit even more efficient. Sitting still for an hour or so should be pretty straightforward if you have feeding to do, so get comfy and enjoy the experience. This can also be good if you're keen to avoid certain hairstyling products for your own sake or the baby's, as you can specify what is used and don't have to breathe in what anyone else is having applied around you. If you find a hairdresser you like and build up a relationship this way it can be good in the long run rather than suddenly finding that your favourite stylist has upped sticks and gone to a new salon miles away.

I think that the most important thing a woman can have – next to talent, of course – is her hairdresser.

Joan Crawford

39

Breathe

THIS MAY SOUND STUPID BUT often we forget to breathe. Yes, air is coming in and going out, but quite possibly in a substandard way, enough to keep us ticking over, not enough to make us feel great when we do it. Many breastfeeding positions can easily lead to a slumped posture (as can so many other activities in life), so take a few moments to get into the habit of good breathing. If you start each feeding session with ten deep, long breaths you will feel better as slow, deep breathing also tends to relax people when they are stressed. So get your shoulders back and your head up, straighten your torso so the air has somewhere to go and get breathing. If you do this every time you feed it will take up a tiny amount of time and you will start to do it at other times too once you know how good it can make you feel.

Breathe. Let go. And remind yourself that this very moment is the only one you know you have for sure.

Oprah Winfrey

40

Watch TV

I USED TO RELIGIOUSLY WATCH THE *Strictly* dance show on TV before I had my first baby. When he came along and I got wrapped up in looking after him I felt like my own life had been swallowed up. But recording and watching back my favourite programmes made me feel like I was back to my own life again. It was only a little thing but the little things can add up, so I'd suggest you plan ahead and set the recorder for whatever programmes you most love. When you're breastfeeding is your chance to watch them back and catch up with soaps, dramas and more. You'll feel like you're getting back some of your small pleasures and also won't feel totally out of the loop when people you're chatting to mention favourite TV programmes and their latest dramatic developments (more on this later). Yes, your older children may insist on their programmes sometimes but you can also introduce them to the delights of your own favourites, for example my little boy was quite taken with *The Great British Bakeoff* cooking show once he realised they were mostly making cakes and biscuits.

I was one of the first generations to watch television. TV exposes people to news, to information, to knowledge, to entertainment. How is it bad?

Tom Clancy

Lose the baby brain

I AM A LITTLE CAUTIOUS OF the phrase 'baby brain'. While I've spoken to plenty of women who say that they felt they couldn't remember anything after having a baby (and sometimes while pregnant too), I feel it is a phrase that gets used to denigrate new mothers and to imply they have somehow become less smart as a result of having a child, which is absurd. A director in the company where I used to work (otherwise a lovely person) told my line manager that I seemed "just the same" in a tone of surprise when I returned to work after having had my first child... why wouldn't I be?! More likely, I think, is that you have quite a lot on your mind and minor things get bumped down the memory list, not to mention that you might be a tad tired and we all know how a lack of sleep affects your brain!

Having said that, I think some women feel their brain *is* going to mush what with sleepless nights and a steep learning curve to contend with and I do also think that there's a tendency towards thinking of nothing *but* the baby, which I think is not always great for your own sense of self and your relationship with others. Hence my cautious use of the phrase for this section, which encourages you to use this wonderful time for thinking and developing yourself mentally.

41

Give your brain
something to work on

Try Sudoku. You might be a genius at this popular number puzzle game or just a beginner. I've been doing them for some time but have never got beyond the easy level – or partway through the intermediate level on a *very* good day. Still, it does make you feel like your brain is working, so it's got to be worth a shot! The American Alzheimer's Association endorsed Sudoku as the kind of brain game that may stave off or improve the onset of the disease. Oh and weirdly, if you have an irritating song stuck in your head and want to get rid of it, the Western Washington University found that doing a (not-too-hard) Sudoku helped! If Sudoku is not for you then try some other brainteasers: crossword puzzles can be fun and of course you can always try one of those 'test your IQ at home' exercises. I came out as a genius on one of those tests, although possibly I forgot to set the timer (ahem).

The problems of puzzles are very near the problems of life.

Erno Rubik

42

Keep a diary

KEEPING A DIARY MAY SOUND like an unthinkable luxury, only for those who can sit back and relax, consider the day's events and then write them down in lovely prose, probably in a leather-bound journal with a fountain pen in exquisite calligraphy. Never mind all that. Get a little notebook and just write one line a day (or even just one word!). There are diaries specially designed for one line a day over the course of five years (so that you can compare year after year) but if that sounds like too much of a commitment then any little notebook will do. If the day's been crap, don't be afraid to say so. If it's been great, revel in it. There will be lots of days that fall in-between these two extremes, but you don't have to write reams, just a little reminder of the day that will probably be interesting to look back on in the future. My mother has kept diaries for years and years and she very kindly lets me read them from time to time – they offer an insight into her as a person that is rare to get on your own mother. You don't have to share your diary of course and most people consider them very private things, but even if it is for your eyes only it can be an insight into your own state of mind and life, which might be hard to get by other means. Look out for patterns emerging, both good and bad, and see if you can improve the bad and get more of the good moments.

I never travel without my diary. One should always have something sensational to read in the train.

Oscar Wilde

43

Memorise a poem

PEOPLE DON'T REALLY DO THIS anymore, but memorising poems used to be something children did quite a lot and so as adults they would have many lovely poems in their memory banks, ready to be taken out and used to entertain themselves and others. I used to sit stony-faced through lots of supposedly sad poems but then wept buckets over one about a little hippopotamus who is disappointed by a birthday present (no idea why, just so *sad!*), so your choice will be very individual to you. If you've not had many dealings with poems until now, get an anthology of popular poems so that you can find a good starting point for your own favourites. Choose a poem you really like (however short) and memorise it. My mother could recite *The Lion and Albert* on long walks, which we children found hilarious. There are dramatic poems and funny poems, tender poems and sad poems, as well as many children's rhyming books which are quite easy to remember after you've read them out loud about a million times. Enjoy the rhymes and rhythms of your favourites and store them in your own memory to keep you company one day or to entertain yourself, friends or children.

Poetry is the spontaneous overflow of powerful feelings.

William Wordsworth

44

Learn a language

CHOOSE A LANGUAGE YOU FEEL the need to refresh or start from scratch with one you've always liked the idea of learning – or perhaps need for work. You'd be surprised how much progress you can make in a very short space of time. My sister went off to South America and did four hours of language classes a day for a month and a half and came back speaking Spanish well enough to comfortably hold a conversation, which improved her CV (for which languages were important), in less than 200 hours. We've already said you may well have more than 700 hours at your disposal while breastfeeding. You can use a language course on a CD or your iPod, add to it by having Skype lessons with a tutor, watch foreign films with subtitles to help you along and listen to foreign language songs – my toddler can sing in Italian despite not knowing the language thanks to a CD of Italian lullabies! All of this can be done while breastfeeding and you could practice your new language skills at local mum and baby sessions for people who speak that language – there may well be one near you. Your new talent could be a great excuse for your next holiday destination and there's nothing like returning to work with a valuable new skill to make you look good!

If you talk to a man in a language he understands, that goes to his head. If you talk to him in his language, that goes to his heart.

Nelson Mandela

45

Do your morning pages

THIS IS AN EXERCISE USED by many writers and in particular recommended by Julia Cameron in her book, *The Artist's Way*. You simply sit down every morning and write three pages. It doesn't matter if they are drivel, it doesn't matter if they are just "I can't think what to write", written over and over again, it doesn't matter if they are rants about the blocked kitchen sink or some other equally irritating small matter. They act as a dumping ground, as a wake-up call, as a warming-up exercise if you have something to write (or other artistic or even non-artistic work to do) and as a slightly crazed diary if that's of interest to you. It seems impossible to fit into a busy life at first if you're not used to it so my advice would be to start small. Get a tiny notepad and do three pages of that, then once you have the habit, upgrade to a slightly bigger one and so on until you're doing 3 A4 sized pages every day. It is a very useful exercise and worth doing even for just a few weeks to see what you think of it.

I started writing morning pages just to keep my hand in, you know, just because I was a writer and I didn't know what else to do but write. And then one day as I was writing, a character came sort of strolling in and I realized, Oh my God, I don't have to be just a screenwriter. I can write novels.

Julia Cameron

46

Write a novel

Always wanted to write a novel or any other piece of writing? Now's your chance. It may sound like madness (as if you don't have enough other stuff to do!), but at least write the first line. The Bulwer-Lytton competition awards a prize to the worst opening line of a novel, so you can amuse yourself by penning a *non*-masterpiece as a starting point. If you happen to come up with something that does actually sound good, then jot down some more thoughts around it and start that novel/short story/textbook/poem/memoir you always meant to write but never quite got round to. If you do some plotting and thinking around it now, then you could always, when you get just a bit more time, enter the National Novel Writing Month event, where your challenge is to knock out the first draft of a novel in one month. Just so you know, this book you are reading was thought of and the basic hundred ideas were written down whilst I was breastfeeding my second child. If I can do it, so can you. Novels, non-fiction, whatever takes your fancy. Just get started. Your morning pages, by the way, are the ideal warm-up exercise for writing a novel.

If you wish to be a writer, write.

Epictetus

47

Take photos

G ET CREATIVE WITH YOUR CAMERA, especially if your phone has a camera, as it can be easier to operate one-handed. Take arty pictures of the room around you, nice photos of your older children playing, cute selfies of yourself and your baby, as well as any other opportunities that crop up: your other half, pets, garden, changes to the house you can tell family and friends about and so on. Now's the time to read the camera manual or at least play with the different settings so you work out what they actually do. I figured out how to take panoramic photos whilst breastfeeding, hence the large number of panoramic pictures of my toes and the room around me on my phone! As you'll be feeding at different times of day you can see how the changing light changes the same shot and you can have fun playing with different adjustments: from filters to altering pictures from colour to black and white and so on. If you take the time to play, you'll be a better photographer after just a few sessions of breastfeeding, as you'll find out what works and what doesn't and why rather than pressing the button and hoping for the best.

Photography is a way of feeling, of touching, of loving. What you have caught on film is captured forever... it remembers little things, long after you have forgotten everything.

Aaron Siskind

48

Expand your knowledge

I S THERE SOMETHING YOU'VE ALWAYS wanted to learn? Perhaps you need to gain a qualification: now could be the time to start, as you're going to have plenty of reading time and more and more educational establishments are offering flexible options to study, from modular learning (you can take several years to get a degree via the Open University if you so wish) to virtual study and correspondence courses. You might just want to get your geography up to speed (my husband despairs of my utter lack of knowledge of which countries sit where on a globe) in which case all you need is a big map pinned up on the wall opposite where you'll be sitting to breastfeed. You might want to become familiar with the work of great artists or your favourite poet. Whatever it is, get started now. Yes, I know you feel horribly busy but even small steps lead to great things and you have an opportunity right now to start that journey. I spent nighttime feeds reading up on the publishing business so that I could understand how best to approach literary agents for traditional publishing as well as how to do self-publishing. It was an education for me and as the books piled up around me I got more confident with my writing plans. Find the gap in your knowledge, however large or small, and fill it.

Education's purpose is to replace an empty mind with an open one.

Malcolm Forbes

49

Do jigsaws

I WAS NEVER MUCH A OF a jigsaw person but now that I have a toddler and he is learning to do jigsaws I find they are quite pleasant to do and fulfilling to achieve (a bit pathetic, I know, to be fulfilled by a 24-piece puzzle). There are puzzles of every level of difficulty and featuring every kind of image. There are even, to my horror, 3D puzzles, which I suspect you will actually need both hands for, so perhaps leave those for later. But having an interesting puzzle on a tray or table next to you can be a good way to while away the time while breastfeeding and you will feel proud when you start doing the more complex ones that you had perhaps never tackled before. To save your sanity, though, can I suggest you don't start off with the thousand piece double-sided ones!

There are no extra pieces in the universe. Everyone is here because he or she has a place to fill, and every piece must fit itself into the big jigsaw puzzle.

Deepak Chopra

50

Read (or listen to) books

I LOVE TO READ BUT GOT busy with my first child and had fallen behind with the latest bestsellers, so when my second baby was born I bought a stash of new novels and enjoyed my nighttime reading sessions. It's surprising how many books you can get through when you're reading for an hour or so every night! Make a list of books you'd love to read or ask people you know for recommendations and get going. Novels are great, books on baby care or baby development can be interesting and useful, how-to and self-help books can tackle parts of your life you always meant to address. If you have an e-reader there are often a lot of promotional deals going so you can fill up your device with good value reads. Your local library is also worth a visit to see what they have that interests you. If you have older children they can enjoy a trip there with you too, while charity shops usually have a lot of cheaply priced books available. If you get really into reading you might also want to join a bookclub: more on this later. If you'd rather lie back with your eyes closed and let someone else read to you (which is quite a nice soothing activity) then consider audio books. There are thousands available so whatever book you'd like to read there's probably an audio book of it available.

Reading is a conversation. All books talk.
But a good book listens as well.

Mark Haddon

51

Cross stitch and crochet

NOPE, I CAN'T DO EITHER of these, or embroider, but while researching this book I came across people suggesting that this was one of the things they could do while breastfeeding. I am in awe. Of course unlike knitting you mostly just need one hand free with the other hand perhaps just holding onto the edge of what you are working on to steady it, so it does make perfect sense. You may be an expert at these crafts already, knocking out the baby hats and decorating nursing cushions like nobody's business, or it may be you are a beginner, in which case having a regular chance to perfect your abilities is great. Start with small and simple things. With cross stitch there are many kits available for the beginner with clear instructions and all the equipment you need while even crocheting simple strips can lead to some very pretty things like decorative flowers.

Love is a canvas furnished by nature and embroidered by imagination.

Voltaire

52

Draw

I was discussing ideas for this book with my artist stepmother, who promptly said: "Drawing" – and she was right of course. If you are of an artistic bent (or always wanted to be) then drawing and indeed painting could be a fantastic thing to do while breastfeeding. Draw what's around you or something from your imagination, practice some aspect of the craft that you've never quite managed to get right or simply enjoy playing with light and shadow, different colours and ideas. You could even draw your own baby as they feed, something of a self-portrait, as part of you will be in there too! For artists who may feel there's no time for their art now that they are juggling children as well, this can be a great way to get back to your calling. If you feel that you can't draw at all then challenge yourself to have a go: steal a child's watercolours or crayons for a little while, get some paper and see what emerges, even if you just have fun turning one colour into another and ending up with muddy brown as you did when you were a child. We all need a bit of playtime.

Drawing makes you see things clearer, and clearer and clearer still, until your eyes ache.

David Hockney

53

Join a bookclub

I BELONG TO A BOOKCLUB MADE up of just five of us, which has been going for many years. Because we live all over town, we usually meet somewhere central, have a nice meal together and discuss the book, as well as many other things along the way. But after each of my two children was born, the bookclub convened at my house one month later, allowing me to feel like I had a social life again, a lovely thing to do for a new mum. You may not already have a bookclub, but if setting one up feels like too much of a commitment right now, you might want to join one online: there are bookclubs on the radio as well as in some newspapers such as *The Guardian*. Much of the work is done for you: a book will be chosen, it is discussed by experts and you the reader can read along and add your comments to the accompanying blog or just read other people's thoughts. It's a nice way to explore a book in more depth than you might usually do and feel part of a wider community of readers. Also, if you are part of a bookclub and accept each book that is chosen, you get to read titles you would never have selected yourself, and this can be very interesting, since everyone tends to get stuck in genre ruts from time to time.

There is more treasure in books than in all the pirate's loot on Treasure Island.

Walt Disney

54

Go to a museum
or art gallery

Not one for every day, but if your baby goes through one of those tedious growth spurts where all they want to do all day is feed, feed, feed, and if you love art then why not settle yourself down for a few hours in a museum or an art gallery (there are usually seats here and there), admire the art and artefacts and let the baby feed away to their belly's content. If you get the chance to do so, total surrendering to their demands during these phases is easier and less stressful than trying to squeeze them in amongst a lot of other things. Also, once sat down, you can admire objects in much more detail than one usually does when conscious of the need to move on to be out of other people's way or to see more items further on. Soak up just a few pieces in all their glory and enjoy the moment, while your breasts get their new orders regarding the quantity of milk to produce. This can be your chance to visit a gallery you've not been to before or a particular show at a museum.

The purpose of art is washing the dust of daily life off our souls.

Pablo Picasso

55

Keep up with the world

MANY OF THE IDEAS IN this book might fall into this category but I feel it's worth re-emphasising. You can feel that your world has shrunk right down to the baby you've just had and nothing else. You may also feel after some time that you've lost touch with some of the interesting things going on in the world and that when you meet old friends and colleagues you have nothing that is not baby-related to talk about, especially with people who do not have children or are not very interested in them. It is easy to talk about nothing but babies when they are taking up all your focus and time and when many of the people you are spending time with (your partner, your NCT group, parents at playgroups you attend) are also caught up with babies. But you are more than your baby and staying in touch with the rest of the world is a good habit to get into. Watch the news from time to time, read the latest bestseller, try out the silly new app that's enjoyably wasting everyone's time, watch that TV show you used to chat to your friends about, stick your nose out of doors and find out what the neighbours are up to or what the weather's like (hard for people like me who prefer to hibernate in winter!). Every conversation you have with someone, make an effort to move on from baby talk after a little while and find out what the other person is up to or discuss something together that is new to both of you. Take a look through the suggestions in this book and find some things you'd enjoy doing while breastfeeding that will make you think about something that is not your baby: have a go at them and feel your world expand a little.

My idea of good company is the company of clever, well-informed people who have a great deal of conversation; that is what I call good company.

Jane Austen

56

Read magazines

MAGAZINES ARE GOOD FOR KEEPING you in touch with things you can't do right now but want to get back to: so I kept up my subscription to *Empire* film magazine while I was on maternity, not because I got to the cinema anything like as often as I'd have liked to but because even reading reviews and interviews was interesting to me and allowed me to keep a mental note of films I wanted to catch up on later. I also took out a subscription to a fashion magazine so I could plan a post-baby wardrobe, which was quite fun when window-shopping was somewhat curtailed by having to take an unenthusiastic toddler with me. Cooking magazines gave me new ideas for recipes to try out at home, parenting magazines can give you good tips and forums to join, travel magazines can give you dreams for your next holiday. You get the idea. Seek out a magazine you'd really like to have and either buy a subscription yourself or ask friends and family for a gift subscription to one or more magazines for your birthday, Christmas or baby shower gifts. Reading a magazine for half an hour can feel like a little bit of luxury in a busy day.

The time to relax is when you don't have time for it.

Sydney J. Harris

57

Open your mind to some new ideas

I LOVE TED, WHICH SHOWCASES INSPIRATIONAL thinkers and leaders from all over the world gathering to talk and share ideas. They have everything from musicians to jugglers, mathematicians to ecologists. The talks last from under five minutes to well over half an hour and make you think about everything from whale poo (really) to inventing new words and everything in between. Give them a go and see what gets you thinking differently or just enjoying something new. It can be quite relaxing to just sit back and listen to some new ideas. I've found things on TED that made me laugh out loud as well as fascinating new data that was useful for my workplace.

This is important: to get to know people, listen, expand the circle of ideas. The world is crisscrossed by roads that come closer together and move apart, but the important thing is that they lead towards the Good.

Pope Francis

58

Tune into the radio

T HE USEFUL THING ABOUT THE radio is it doesn't need any hands at all and doesn't even require you to look at it, so if you'd just like to lie back and close your eyes while feeding your baby, this could be the medium for you. Many people have their own favourite programmes such as long-running soap operas or *Woman's Hour*, but there may be many aspects of radio you haven't yet explored: new dramas and wonderfully re-told classics, bookclubs, the news, cookery shows, comedy and of course music of every kind. You may have got stuck in a rut, always listening to the same radio stations, so branch out a little. Or radio generally may be quite new to you because you're more used to other forms of media, in which case it's a whole new world to explore. If you get into the radio you can also look out for podcasts from various sources as again, you can just lie back and listen.

It's not true I had nothing on, I had the radio on.

Marilyn Monroe

Make time for your older children

Having a second child raises the whole issue of sibling jealousy. However kind and understanding your older child is, they are bound to feel a bit left out at certain times and one of those times is when you are breastfeeding your new baby. It is an obviously intimate and cosy moment between you and the new arrival, which can lead to jealousy and therefore bad behaviour from your older child as they seek to draw your attention to themselves instead of their sibling. This of course is rather irritating when you feel like you are already giving quite a lot to a child at that moment, so you may not respond well to the attention-seeking behaviour and thus quite possibly make it worse.

Head trouble off at the pass by finding ways to give attention to your older child while your baby feeds. This section offers some good ways to spend time with your older children while breastfeeding, which I hope will keep everyone happy.

59

Read together

" I've got an arm free," I say enticingly to my toddler while I am breastfeeding. "Come and have a hug and I'll read to you." He turns the pages while I read to (and hug) him, a cosy moment with both my children. I have always loved reading to him and this is a good time to share together, especially as breastfeeding can arouse jealousy in older children – here is the tiny baby being cuddled and given sustenance and what are they getting? A hug and a shared story can be a comfort to them at this moment. Your baby is also getting the benefit of hearing stories, rhymes and the rhythm of reading. So keep a stack of favourite stories by your feeding stations and offer story time at the same time as feeding time: it is often welcomed. If your child does not like it at first, persevere. My little boy initially refused, I think he felt it would not be the same with a baby hogging the main seat but now that he is used to the new arrangement he enjoys it.

Storytelling is a very old human skill that gives us an evolutionary advantage. If you can tell young people how you kill an emu, acted out in song or dance, or that Uncle George was eaten by a croc over there, don't go there to swim, then those young people don't have to find out by trial and error.

Margaret Atwood

60

Take part in their
play – vocally

I T'S SURPRISING BUT OFTEN WHAT a child really wants is for
you to just be present when they are playing. So you don't
actually need to be down on all fours building a new Thomas
railway track or helping Teddy onto the bus: you can simply sit
nearby and comment. Ask questions about the game, suggest
activities for characters, sing along with songs or make important
announcements: "Red light – everyone STOP! Green light – off
you go!" Your child will probably enjoy this and feel that although
you may be feeding the baby your attention is actually on them. So
don't feel like you must be physically involved to be playing with
your older child – give them your focus and they will be happy.

It should be noted that children at play are not playing about; their games should be seen as their most serious-minded activity.

Michel de Montaigne

61

Supervise activities

I F YOU KNOW A FEED is coming up, you can arrange activities for your older child. Jigsaws (which you can help with), play dough, drawing and so on can all be good things to arrange beforehand, avoiding your child suddenly getting bored just as you need to breastfeed and then causing chaos while you look on helplessly. I would suggest though that if you're setting up an activity it will make your life easier if it's something relatively clean. Now is not the best time to get out the watercolours or suggest making mud pies! Stacking games, playing 'postman' with a cardboard box and some old envelopes and so on are all good games for this.

You see a child play, and it is so close to seeing an artist paint, for in play a child says things without uttering a word. You can see how he solves his problems. You can also see what's wrong. Young children, especially, have enormous creativity, and whatever's in them rises to the surface in free play.

Erik Erikson

62

Watch movies together

IF YOU CAN WREST YOUR children away from their obsessive
favourites (Thomas the Tank Engine, Peppa Pig and more) for
a short while, then you can introduce them to new films that you
can share together. My toddler likes dancing about in muddy
puddles, so I showed him the famous dance sequence from the
film *Singin' in the Rain* and was rewarded a week later when I
saw him singing the song while splashing about in the garden
on a wet day, melting my heart as he did so. For very little
ones find some shorter films and animations, for the older ones
perhaps introduce them to something more demanding from the
pantheon of children's classics. If you are sitting by them you can
help the narration along in any hard-to-understand moments or
provide reassurance during mildly scary parts and see them enjoy
the same films you did as a child or find some new favourites.
Either way you will have fun and spend some time together.

As I get older, I want to do more films for kids because they're the best audience around. Just putting a smile on a kid's face is the best thing.

James McAvoy

63

List good things about your children

I ONCE READ AN INTERESTING ARTICLE about your children and having favourites. The point made was that you *love* them all the same but might not always *like* them all the same, as each of them in turn tries your patience or is particularly enchanting. Your new baby may be tiny, quiet, needing little input and very sweet, meanwhile your toddler may be pushing every one of your buttons to get attention, requiring huge amounts of input and frequently doing unappealing things like keeping one finger permanently up their nose. You may love them both/all fiercely but it can be easy to like your new baby more on certain occasions. Look hard at your older child and remind yourself how clever they are, how exciting it is that they can talk and do amazing new things every day, how beautiful they are and how enthusiastic they can be about all sorts of things and so on. The liking will come back. No doubt when your sweet baby hits the Terrible Twos and your older child is more reasonable and being (mostly) charming to you the balance will tip again and you will have to remind yourself that you do actually like your screaming toddler too. Take some time to remind yourself (especially on the days when they are driving you nuts) why both you love *and* like your children and what you find wonderful about each of them, especially the ones who are being most difficult.

Children will not remember you for the material things you provided but for the feeling that you cherished them

Richard L. Evans

64

Escape to the park

I F STAYING INDOORS IS DRIVING you and the kids nuts and you are lucky enough to have a park nearby then decamp there to feed on a day when your baby wants to stay attached to you like a limpet for hours at a time. Your older ones can run about, you can get on with breastfeeding. Wrap up warm, this might get cold in the winter months, but a bit of fresh air will blow the cobwebs away and on a sunny day it will be a very pleasant experience. For extra fun you can always commandeer one of the larger swings at the playground for yourself.

When was the last time you spent a quiet moment just doing nothing – just sitting and looking at the sea, or watching the wind blowing the tree limbs, or waves rippling on a pond, a flickering candle or children playing in the park?

Ralph Marston

65

Play board games

IF YOUR OTHER CHILDREN ARE old enough then board games can be quite appealing. You can easily play a game with them one-handed (they may even want to throw the dice for you!) and it's a good time to show them new games they've not yet played. My toddler got introduced to Four-in-a-Row, Snakes and Ladders and Ludo and was very interested in finding out about rules and new actions like shaking and throwing dice (halfway across the room, mostly) as well as quickly discovering how to cheat!

I like to play board games a lot with my girl, things like that. We attempt to cook. And even if it goes wrong, it doesn't matter because it's the time you spend doing it that's important.

Sam Worthington

66

Sing

CRANK UP THE MUSIC AND sing with your children while you feed. Nursery rhymes and songs are good for this and they can dance about to any that take their fancy while you join in with the singing. It's an easy way to take part since you don't need your voice while feeding and they can feel that you are involved. If they're older and homework is due you could always resort to educational songs like the Disco Times Tables I had as a child... hideous 'tunes' (if you can call them that) but still very memorable to this day!

Music is the greatest communication in the world. Even if people don't understand the language that you're singing in, they still know good music when they hear it.

Lou Rawls

Stay in touch with your friends and family

THE BUSYNESS OF BEING A new parent (even second or more times round, if anything more so) can tend to leave your connections dangling. You don't have as much time or energy to go out, so people tend to come to you (which is not that fair after a while), you can't stay up late because you're knackered and you aren't replying to emails and other forms of communication. It's all too easy to allow your friends and family to slip away just at the time when you need them most and want to speak to someone in something other than baby talk. Taking into account your new limitations, you need to find some ways to keep in touch. Of course try and find opportunities to go out and socialise, but while you're breastfeeding you can at least use the time to keep friendships and family ties ticking over, ready for the next time you can meet in person.

67

Get texting

BACK TO THE *STRICTLY* TV dance show – before babies, my sister and I would watch the show together sometimes and avidly discuss it when we were apart. I thought I'd lost that link when my little one came along but my sister is an avid texter and I found myself texting back and forth with her during the live show while I breastfed – commenting on each dance, the costumes, gossip we'd picked up from somewhere, the scores and much more. It was only for an hour or so once a week but it was fun and made it feel like she was in the room with me, an easy way to share something. My brother is not one for writing long letters or emails but he does love photo messages, so he'll regularly text me images of everything from the floor tiles in the house he is renovating to the family dog making a funny face. It's a little moment from his everyday life and I respond in kind with pictures of my children playing or the garden on a sunny day. Communication doesn't have to be about the big things, it can just be the tiny moments that make up your life and keep you in the loop with someone else's.

My cell phone is my best friend. It's my lifeline to the outside world.

Carrie Underwood

68

Pick up the phone

SOMETIMES YOU NEED TO ACTUALLY hear someone's voice and have a longer catch-up to feel connected. When this happens, pick up the phone and actually call your friend – this is becoming a rare thing nowadays but it doesn't need to be! Texting is great for quick messages but if something bigger or more emotional is happening it can be good to hear the other person's voice and judge how they are feeling for yourself: emoticons don't always have the answer! Find out what are good days or times to call or just pick up the phone to say you are thinking of someone. My husband and I have a pretty regular midday chat when he is at work, it doesn't last more than a few minutes but it's a way of touching base and knowing how the other person's day is going.

That's the sign of a good relationship, when you can pick up a phone and it doesn't matter when the last time you spoke was.

Joe Torre

69

Set up video messaging

I F YOU'RE UNLIKELY TO BE able to see your friend in person any time soon then using Skype or other video messaging services is a good idea. When I had my first child, so did one of my closest friends – but she had just moved to France during her maternity leave and I missed her. We Skyped while breastfeeding, laughing over our ludicrously enhanced breasts and very nearly crying over our combined lack of sleep. It was a great way to feel connected and 'see' each other when distance didn't permit dropping round for a cup of tea and meant that a year later when she returned to the UK we didn't feel like we'd lost all that time out of our friendship. This kind of communication can be good for your older kids too: my toddler loves to see his grandparents on Skype. So if your friends or family are long-distance a lot of the time then get into the habit of video messaging, perhaps setting up a regular weekend call or a time of day when you know you have a long feeding session ahead of you.

We FaceTime and Skype. My two older kids got iPods for their birthdays, so they can FaceTime their dad whenever they need him. They always get a six o'clock call right after dinner, and I make sure I talk to each child. Even my 1-year-old gets on the phone and says 'Daddy.'

CC Sabathia

70

Use your favourite
social media

I WON'T EVEN LIST ALL THE different kinds of social media you could be using to keep up with your friends and family, as they'll be out of date by the time this is published, so let's just say that whatever kinds of social media you enjoy the most, use them to keep up with your friends and their lives. I would say that some social media can feel a little 'removed', however it's a good stop-gap and as many people nowadays announce quite important things online (engagements, pregnancies, babies, new houses and jobs) before telling people face to face, it's worth keeping up! This one is excellent for middle-of-the-night communication as you won't be disturbing anyone! If you're not using any kind of social media at all, perhaps try one or two sites and find out what the majority of your friends are using so that you can find them easily once you get started.

Social media allows me to pick my times for social interaction.

Guy Kawasaki

71

Write a letter or card

B ECAUSE WE USE SOCIAL MEDIA and phones so much, the art of letter writing is fading away. But people still really like getting cards, letters and postcards through the door instead of the usual junk, so perhaps you could buck the trend. Buy up a stash of silly, amusing or heartfelt postcards and drop your friends a line from time to time so that they know you're still thinking of them even if you're perhaps not seeing them as often as you used to. You may feel like contact and communication is an all or nothing affair, but it really isn't. I have a friend who doesn't often write, but he will always come and see me when he's in town, which is very touching to me because I know that he still thinks of me even if there's no word from him for a while. So don't feel that your friends will have forgotten you just because you're a little out of circulation: drop them a line and let them know you'll be back soon.

I love the rebelliousness of snail mail, and I love anything that can arrive with a postage stamp. There's something about that person's breath and hands on the letter.

Diane Lane

72

Breastfeed as a group

THIS IS ONE THAT WORKS well if you have local friends with children of the same age. If you've joined the NCT, for example, you'll end up with a group of perhaps seven other mums all with babies exactly the same age as yours. So if you have a day where your baby wants constant feeding and so do theirs, meet up and do the feeding together. Being parked on the sofa for much of the day is more fun with someone to chat to. Even if it's just your baby (or just theirs) then invite yourself round or ask them over so that you can make your feeding a more social event.

Any time women come together with a collective intention, it's a powerful thing. Whether it's sitting down making a quilt, in a kitchen preparing a meal, in a club reading the same book, or around the table playing cards, or planning a birthday party, when women come together with a collective intention, magic happens.

Phylicia Rashad

Stay in love with
your partner

THE ARRIVAL OF CHILDREN CAN be hard on your connection to your partner. You have a new person on whom to focus your love and attention and you may be tired and irritable with your partner, as they may be with you. You may well feel 'touched out' from holding a baby all the time and having them breastfeed from you and not feel like having anyone else touch you, sexually or otherwise. Your conversation with one another may become limited to information on how many poos the baby has done today and whose turn it is to change the nappy. None of this is helpful to a relationship. This section focuses on a few small ways in which you can hold on to that connection while breastfeeding and keep it going until it can once again claim some time, space and energy back for itself. Hang on in there, it does get better!

73

Take time to talk and cuddle

IT'S EASY FOR YOUR PARTNER to see your feeding time as you being 'busy' but really, this is an excellent time for you to sit together and chat about anything and everything. It gives you quiet and uninterrupted time together, which is lovely when you are otherwise busy. If you have older children, see if you can get them to do 'quiet time', where they play by themselves for a little while: this is a good habit for them to learn anyway and gives you some quality time with your partner. If they are too young for this, then set them up with some nice things to do (see earlier section) and enjoy shared family time. If you can sit in a position where you are cuddled up together with your partner, even better, so that you are getting some touching time that does not mean anything sexual is expected but is simply enjoying being close together.

Too often we underestimate the power of a touch, a smile, a kind word, a listening ear, an honest compliment, or the smallest act of caring, all of which have the potential to turn a life around.

Leo Buscaglia

74

Plan something nice
for your partner

I F YOU WANT TO KEEP the flame burning with your partner, then a good idea is to spend your breastfeeding time to plan something special for them. Perhaps an outing for both of you *sans* baby, or a 'birthday book' with contributions from family and friends. I developed a list of 40 things for my husband to do for his 40th birthday and most of the list was composed during breastfeeding sessions, as I scribbled down ideas and then researched options for activities and experiences. They will be touched by the fact that despite your busy life and having a lot of other plates to juggle you have still taken the time to think of their needs and what would make them happy. And you may find your thoughtfulness being reciprocated.

We've got this gift of love, but love is like a precious plant. You can't just accept it and leave it in the cupboard or just think it's going to get on by itself. You've got to keep watering it. You've got to really look after it and nurture it.

John Lennon

75

Study the Kama Sutra

Sex may be the last thing on your mind on some days (weeks, months…) but one thing you can do is return to the marital bed a little more adventurous and knowledgeable than when you left it: quality does count for something when quantity and opportunities decrease. Get a copy of the Kama Sutra or a similar book and find something new to introduce in future romantic moments with your partner. Your partner will no doubt be surprised and pleased and you will feel less like a worn out mummy and more of a sex goddess than you perhaps expected. It only takes a few moments to get some new ideas and it could make a difference to your sex life, so it's worth the effort. And whatever the outcome of your new moves, the fact that you've made the effort in the first place will make you partner feel good.

Love is an ice cream sundae, with all the marvellous coverings. Sex is the cherry on top.

Jimmy Dean

76

Ask your partner to give you a massage

I'VE ALREADY SAID THAT YOU can easily end up without much physical contact between you and your partner in the early and most tiring days, so even if a full-body sensual massage with candles, oils and romantic music is out, ask your partner to give you a hand or foot massage while you are feeding. It may only take a few minutes but it does make a difference. You will feel pampered and your partner will feel appreciated, as you are likely to be grateful and pleased in a way that you probably don't express when they change a nappy or load the dishwasher. The physical contact is also important between both of you and will do a lot for your relationship in the short term.

Touch seems to be as essential as sunlight.

Diane Ackerman

77

List good things about your partner

JUST AS WITH YOUR OLDER children, you may find it hard to recall why it is that you still love this person who has not changed as many nappies as you'd like or is irritating you by sleeping soundly through yet *another* midnight feed. Take some time to remember how you met, fell in love, your time together before children and your partner's good qualities as a parent. Recall the ways in which they support you on a day-to-day basis as much as in the big things in life and focus on the good feelings you have about them engendered by this exercise. Undertake to do this regularly, because the early days of parenthood are hard on a relationship and it needs all the help it can get. It is all too easy to drift into being slightly irritated by each other most of the time and forget that these small irritations are not who either of you really are. Many of your arguments or annoyances are probably caused by sleep deprivation anyway, so don't let them hurt a good partnership. You can ask your partner to do the same for you, so that both of you are focusing on the good in each other at least some of the time.

You learn to speak by speaking, to study by studying, to run by running, to work by working; in just the same way, you learn to love by loving.

Anatole France

78

Play together

D IG OUT A BOARD GAME: anything will do from Scrabble to Snakes and Ladders. Set it up and play with your partner while you are breastfeeding. It'll be silly and funny and will have you talking about something that isn't the baby (however lovely they are). You can pick up where you left off if your feed comes to an end before the game does and meanwhile recapture some 'couple' time on a small scale. Add silly rules if it makes it more 'your' game, such as bonus points for rude words in Scrabble or reversing the effects of ladders and snakes. Whatever makes the experience fun and memorable is great and will make you both feel a little more connected and less 'just parents'.

Mix a little foolishness with your serious plans. It is lovely to be silly at the right moment.

Horace

Multitask to free
up more time

B REASTFEEDING HAS SOME LIMITATIONS IN terms of what you can get done, being more or less one-handed. But it does give you time, which is precious in the horribly busy life that is the lot of all parents, and so this section offers a few ideas for multitasking. Get some of the must-do things off your list while breastfeeding, leaving you with more time to do nice-to-do things once you've finished or just to feel that you are vaguely on top of things again. I'm sure you do a lot of these things naturally, but here are a few reminders of what you could be doing to free up your time.

79

Write emails

I BET YOU HAVE EMAILS STACKED up in your inbox and feel bad about not getting round to answering them, whether from friends, work, domestic tasks or whatever else. Take the opportunity to a) unsubscribe from anything you no longer want to receive (this usually needs doing every few months to get rid of all the annoying junk mail) and b) answer just one or two easy ones. If you have lots of family/friends asking how you're doing, send pictures, it can be quicker and easier than a long-winded (and possibly dull) daily account of your life, as well as cuter! Without lots of itsy bitsy emails hanging around you'll have a chance to get round to the more complicated ones when you have some headspace clear for them. A one-page inbox (no scrolling!) is quite a restful sight. If you can't give a proper answer to something then send a holding email to say you'll get back to someone so that at least you don't feel hounded or guilty.

It is while you are patiently toiling at the little tasks of life that the meaning and shape of the great whole of life dawn on you.

Phillips Brooks

80

Write to-do lists

I AM AN INVETERATE LIST-MAKER, SO I always have a notepad somewhere nearby with long lists of things to do scribbled all over its pages. Some get done, others don't, but writing things down can mean that you are reminded of their importance as well as getting the satisfaction of crossing them off when they're done. It also means letting go of them from inside your brain, so if you're one of those people who can't get back to sleep after a night feed because things are rushing around in your head, then writing them down on a piece of paper may help you get a better night's rest. Most of my nighttime feeds result in scribbled notes to myself, which get read (if legible) in the morning and acted on without me having to try and recall them after a bad night's sleep. Your to-do list can be everything from the day-to-day stuff to the more adventurous: from changing the cat litter to ideas for a great holiday.

Women in particular need to keep an eye on their physical and mental health, because if we're scurrying to and from appointments and errands, we don't have a lot of time to take care of ourselves. We need to do a better job of putting ourselves higher on our own 'to do' list.

Michelle Obama

81

Do your shopping online

THIS ONE IS A NO-BRAINER. If you have a family then I guarantee you don't really have time to wander about a supermarket and then lug everything home, all the while fending off the pleading of older children who have spotted some treat they'd really like to have. Get an online shopping account set up with your favourite retailer (they all seem to have a home delivery service now) and book a time slot that suits your lifestyle. We used to have ours come after the kids were in bed but now we've realised it is a source of much interest and entertainment for our toddler, so now it arrives as a post-nursery 'treat' in the middle of the afternoon and we have a willing if slightly worryingly keen helper (don't let them carry the eggs, is all I'm saying). When you're all set up you can do your weekly shop while you breastfeed, thus effectively feeding the whole family at one stroke. Once you're doing your grocery shop online, why not shop for everything else online too? Even if you like to support small businesses, most of these also have an online presence nowadays, so you can still buy from your favourite companies. My second child was born two months before Christmas and all my festive shopping, gifts and cards got done online that year! There are even companies who will wrap your gifts and send them directly to the recipient, saving you time and hassle wrapping and trudging to the post office. You can create and send personalised cards to people, sort out your holidays, do your banking online and so much more. If you have not yet fully embraced online shopping, now might be the time to get into it: it will save you a lot of time just when you most need it in your life. If you're already an online shopping expert, take a look and see what else can be done online that you have not yet explored.

Melissa Addey

The secret of getting things done is to act!

Dante Alighieri

82

Keep up with your correspondence

F ROM CHRISTMAS CARDS TO NEW baby cards to thank you cards (there's a lot of those to write after a new baby comes along and everyone sends you lovely things for them), birthday cards and cards for just about every other occasion, breastfeeding can be a good time to keep up with your correspondence if you get yourself set up right. Have a collection of nice cards prepared and sit by a table to feed, allowing you (at least while your baby drinks on one side) to fulfil some of your social obligations quickly and easily. You can use companies like Vistaprint or others to order your own cards ready-personalised, saving on some of the repetitive parts of writing, for example a standard Christmas greeting and your family's names ready-written, leaving you to write something more personal to the recipient.

Make it a habit to tell people thank you. To express your appreciation, sincerely and without the expectation of anything in return. Truly appreciate those around you, and you'll soon find many others around you. Truly appreciate life, and you'll find that you have more of it.

Ralph Marston

83

Update your technology

Now is the time to say "yes" when your computer asks if it can update your software. It's the time to install and programme new software and apps that can do everything from satellite navigation (no more getting lost or rows in the car over map-reading) to planning meetings and social occasions, set up live bus arrival times for your local bus stops, diary reminder entries for everyone's birthdays and arrange text alerts from your bank before you go overdrawn. It's the time to find a game that will entertain your toddler and download it to your phone and the time to update your contact lists and address book. Or just have fun 'training' your voice recognition software. These are the boring little things we never get round to but then wish we had because they make our lives smoother, quicker and better informed. So set up those downloads and settle back to feed while they do their thing. You'll be glad of them later.

The number one benefit of information technology is that it empowers people to do what they want to do. It lets people be creative. It lets people be productive. It lets people learn things they didn't think they could learn before, and so in a sense it is all about potential.

Steve Ballmer

84

Express milk

Y OU MAY NEED TO EXPRESS milk to feed your baby with a
bottle for occasions such as covering your working hours,
going out for social occasions and so on, or possibly to help with
encouraging production or easing issues like mastitis. Expressing
from one side while you feed on the other (if your baby does not
take both sides at a feed) will probably be a good use of time as
your let-down reflex will work better when your baby is right
there suckling from you. Expressing can be a bit slow and tedious
to do, so combining feeding and expressing can be a good use of
your time.

The more people have studied different methods of bringing up children the more they have come to the conclusion that what good mothers and fathers instinctively feel like doing for their babies is the best after all.

Benjamin Spock

85

Plan meals for the week

STANDING IN FRONT OF CUPBOARDS and fridges pondering
what to make for each meal gets boring and doesn't really
inspire creative solutions. Making a meal planner for the week
means your shopping will be more efficiently tailored to what
you are actually going to use and means you will always know
what you're supposed to be cooking (you can switch meals round
if you don't fancy what's on the menu that day!). I have a blank
one-page sheet with a table that contains the date/days of the
week and Breakfast/Lunch/Supper for each as well as space for
notes, e.g. someone coming to lunch. I fill it in once a week
and then do the shopping. The list then gets stuck up in the
kitchen and solves meal dilemmas for the rest of the week. At the
bottom, we scribble things we've run out of for next week's shop.
It saves a lot of time and energy as well as allowing us to plan
ahead and introduce interesting new meals to try on appropriate
days like the weekends when everyone has a bit more time for
experimenting. Make your own little sheet and use the time while
breastfeeding to create your menu for the week: you'll have nicer
food and spend less time worrying about what to make.

I think careful cooking is love, don't you? The loveliest thing you can cook for someone who's close to you is about as nice a valentine as you can give.

Julia Child

86

Do your work prep

YOU MAY HAVE GONE BACK to work and still be breastfeeding, in which case this is a good time to catch up on papers that need to be read, exams that need to be marked, presentations that need to be given and so on. Practice your speech to your audience of one, review conversations you need to have and plan for your annual appraisal. Make the most of this quiet time to get the boring work things done and dusted so that when you've finished a feed and are two-handed again you can enjoy doing something non work-related.

The best preparation for good work tomorrow is to do good work today.

Elbert Hubbard

87

Run your own business

I RECENTLY MET UP WITH A business consultant who said he'd already seen the new baby of an entrepreneur friend of mine – before I had – he'd attended a business meeting that the baby had shown up for! Little babies will quite happily feed or sleep their way through business meetings so there's no reason not to take them along if you run your own company or if you have a forward-thinking workplace, especially in the early days (later on, when they start chewing your paper supply and randomly phoning clients while playing with your phones, this strategy might need a re-think...). If you work from home, even better, as the baby will not be a distraction to anyone else and you can make phone calls, type one-handed and look things up on the internet while your baby is otherwise happily engaged.

Entrepreneurship isn't for everyone, and not everyone is going to be an entrepreneur, but women who turn to business, turn to economics, because there are people depending on them, I think that their creativity, their resilience, their spirit, embody what's best about entrepreneurship.

Gayle Tzemach Lemmon

88

Get to grips with
your paperwork

W HEN'S THE LAST TIME YOU actually looked at your bank
statement properly? Take this time to sit and look through
it in detail. You'll notice anything untoward more quickly if
it happens (e.g. people using your cards), realise bad spending
habits – my husband pointed out that little 'top-up' shops at the
supermarket were adding up to a few hundred a year – and avoid
bank charges like overdraft usage if you make a few changes to
how you manage your money. Also take a moment to check on
things like the list of direct debits you have and cancel any that
are no longer of benefit, like gym memberships you don't use or
magazines you are no longer interested in. You'll be surprised
how poring over a boring piece of paper can reap real financial
rewards from time to time. What other paperwork has been
hanging about for ages? It took my husband and me over three
years to make a will after the birth of our first child but we finally
contacted a legal firm and were sent questionnaires to fill in as a
first step. Use the feeding time to scribble down your answers and
make notes about anything you need to find out or provide so
that you are one step closer to getting your will completed. If you
die without a will your possessions may not be distributed as you
wished. If you are unmarried your partner may not inherit from
you at all and vice versa, possibly causing serious problems. If you
have children, you need to specify who will care for them and so
on. If you have already made a will and your circumstances since
then have changed (e.g. getting married) your existing will could
be rendered null and void. So it's worth doing, however tedious it
may seem. Having got underway with that, we're now looking at
life insurance. Seems like there's always something!

In all affairs it's a healthy thing now and then to hang a question mark on the things you have long taken for granted.

Bertrand Russell

89

Sort out your photos

WE'RE TAKING MORE PHOTOS THAN ever because we have cameras built into our phones and our cameras are digital so we don't feel like we are using up expensive film. But do these photos ever get seen again? This can be a good time to transfer your photos onto the computer (at the last count my phone had something absurd like 800 photos on it), sort them into files and choose ones to print. You can then upload them to photo sites (I've used various including Photo Box) where they will be printed and posted back to you in a matter of days. You won't believe how many photos you take of a newborn, so this could be a good activity after a few months have gone by! Many sites also now make really nice printed photo albums. I made one for my first baby and am halfway through one for my second: again, find a photo site, upload the photos you want to use, have fun arranging them in a book (there are lots of different layouts to choose from) and then sit back and wait for a lovely professional-looking album to drop through your letterbox. These albums make a great gift for new grandparents and my toddler is very proud of 'his' book.

Photography to me is catching a moment which is passing, and which is true.

Jacques-Henri Lartigue

Rethink and revamp your life

YOUR LIFE WILL HAVE BEEN thrown up, down and all around by your new, small arrival. So take a moment to see whether there is any part of your life that needs rethinking and revamping. It's interesting to me how many women change their career paths entirely when they have a baby and I believe this is because you get new priorities and perspectives that arrive along with the baby. Breastfeeding, by giving you time to sit and think for a while, can give you a valuable opportunity to reflect on your changed life and change it even further according to your new focus. Take a moment to dream.

90

Follow your dreams

MY DREAM IS TO BE a full-time writer. While my first child napped, I wrote a novel. With my second baby, as I breastfed, I wrote the notes that made up the book you're reading now. I grabbed every feeding chance I got to move closer to my dream of being a writer. So if I can write a book while breastfeeding (and I assure you I am not a superwoman by any stretch of the imagination), what would you like to do? Take some time to focus on what your dreams and goals are and then use your breastfeeding time to get one tiny step closer to them. It doesn't matter if it's just a little move forwards, it's a move all the same and you might be surprised at what it leads on to. Also, it's a funny thing, but often once you've focused on a goal, opportunities seem to present themselves to help you move towards achieving it, perhaps simply because you notice them more. So sit and daydream for a while, then identify your own dreams and think of what you can do while breastfeeding to make them happen.

You can't put a limit on anything. The
more you dream, the farther you get.

Michael Phelps

91

Get more creative

THINK OF YOUR BRAIN LIKE lots of little paths. If you think about going to work your brain will just go down its usual 'route' of whatever your normal way to work consists of. But if you think of a new way to go to work your brain will need to create a new pathway to take account of this new and surprising change. It's easy to let your thinking get routine, so a simple way to get more creative is to do routine things differently. Add an unusual new ingredient to a salad, read a magazine or paper you would never usually read or take a new route to a well-known destination: my toddler nearly had a nervous breakdown when I tried this going to the park, so clearly his brain route was already firmly fixed. Listen to music that is not your usual taste or watch a film you wouldn't usually pick and so on. You'll find over time that you will start to think of new ideas, make different connections and perhaps change your mind about a few things of which you were certain. Creativity is yours for the asking: just act differently.

Creativity is just connecting things. When you ask creative people how they did something, they feel a little guilty because they didn't really do it, they just saw something. It seemed obvious to them after a while. That's because they were able to connect experiences they've had and synthesize new things.

Steve Jobs

92

Plan a new wardrobe

A FTER ALMOST A YEAR WEARING less than flattering maternity wear (seriously, retailers need to do some more work on their maternity wear offerings), you may be desperate not just to get back to your own clothes but to have a whole new you emerge, butterfly-like, from the cocoon of your maternity wardrobe. This may be especially true when you feel that you have completed your childbearing efforts and are entering a new stage of your life. So grab some fashion magazines and browse your favourite clothes and shoe shops online to see what they have to offer. Choose a new wardrobe, or at least a few items that will make you feel great. If you're not in a hurry you can get great bargains on eBay and outlet sites for your favourite brands as you will know what size you are. I spent several months slowly amassing items that I loved and wanted so that when I got (some of) my figure back and no longer needed nursing-friendly tops I had some really lovely things to wear. You could even use Pinterest to create a mood board of ideas for your new style.

You have a more interesting life if you wear impressive clothes.

Vivienne Westwood

93

Change the way you eat

Y OUR FIRST THOUGHT ON THIS subject may be "lose weight" but this has to be approached gently as a very low-calorie diet is not recommended while you are breastfeeding. Instead, introduce some good healthy new habits now such as eating a little less meat, a lot more fruit and vegetables, adding nuts and good quality dairy (or equivalent changes if you are vegetarian/ vegan) to your diet and getting plenty of water to drink. Make sure you eat breakfast, manage your snack intake (enough to keep you going but not too many... goodbye beloved biscuits, sigh...) and encourage the whole family to eat new and varied meals. Revamping your meals can be interesting as we all get stuck in cooking ruts, so get hold of a few new recipe books or look online and jot down different ideas. This can also be good for getting older children to be more adventurous in their food choices. You can plan longer-term how to lose any excess weight you may have put on but the small changes you make to eat more healthily and adventurously may help with that without you even realising it, until the scales surprise you in a good way!

Melissa Addey

Food, in the end, in our own tradition, is something holy. It's not about nutrients and calories. It's about sharing. It's about honesty. It's about identity.

Louise Fresco

94

Plan and research

THERE ARE SO MANY THINGS that need planning or researching in life. Finding and buying a house, finding childcare or schools for your children, developing new ideas for work and home, finding out if there is a car-sharing service near you: whatever it is that needs doing in your life, use this time to do your planning and research. It's good thinking time too, if you need to weigh up one choice over another. Use this time wisely and you'll find yourself getting more done that you'd believe possible.

Planning is bringing the future into the present so that you can do something about it now.

Alan Lakein

95

Declutter

W E COULD ALL DO WITH a sort-out from time to time as we accumulate too much stuff or the wrong stuff for where we're at in our lives. You may think you need two hands for this job and you sort of do, but it depends on what you are intent on decluttering. I went through my jewellery collection (sadly I seem a bit short on the diamonds front...) and tidied it all up, which only required one hand. But my top tip for this activity is that you sit down opposite something that needs sorting and just stare at it while you are feeding the baby. Sort it mentally. It's the mental sorting of objects that takes time, not the physical side. Look at a bookcase for a while and choose ten books that need to move along to a new home: perhaps to friends or a charity shop. When you get up from the breastfeeding, it will take you all of one minute to take the books off the shelf and stick them in a bag, because you've already done the mental sorting. You could sell on your unwanted items and buy something to make yourself feel good, for example new clothing or music. This works for books, CDs, DVDs, children's toys which frequently need re-sorting, wardrobes (just leave the doors open) and so on.

Melissa Addey

When we clear the physical clutter from our lives, we literally make way for inspiration and 'good, orderly direction' to enter.

Julia Cameron

96

Write a bucket list

Y OU MAY BE FEELING A little constrained in some ways: for starters you're one-handed while breastfeeding, not to mention your lovely new baby may have turned your usual world and routine topsy-turvy. I know both of mine did. So why not write yourself a 'bucket list' of things you'd like to do once you get some things back: your two hands, a good night's sleep, the odd night out, perhaps even a weekend away. It will highlight the things you miss the most from your former life and you can take steps towards getting them back into your life as soon as possible. It doesn't all have to be swimming with dolphins either, it can be spending more time with loved ones or time alone, time to reflect on your life or anything else that you feel would make you happy and that you need to focus on to bring into your life.

Melissa Addey

People talk about this 'bucket list': 'I need to go to this country, I need to skydive.' Whereas I need to think as much as I can, to feel as much as I can, to be conscious and observe and understand me and the people around me as much as I can.

Amy Tan

97

(Re)Design your house

Again: use your 'looking' time to figure out the details of whatever changes you want to make to your house: whether it's just a new shade of paint or a serious piece of renovation or restructuring, the time you spend thinking is really the hard part. Getting on with it afterwards will be much easier once you've really thought through what you want and how you want it done. Spending thinking time on it upfront will mean you understand what you actually want from your home and how to achieve it – which may be easier than you think: sometimes it's a case of de-cluttering (see earlier), a change of use for an item or even a room rather than wholesale changes or expansion that are needed.

I think taking design out of the studio and really having a relationship with the people that you're making it for really convinced me of how powerful a thing design is. It's not just an aesthetic decoration.

Genevieve Gorder

98

Plan a holiday

U SE THE TIME YOU HAVE while feeding your baby – and a computer if there's one handy – to plan your next holiday. It may be your first family holiday (two words of advice: baby wipes) or your first break as a couple since having kids, but you can find the perfect place and do all the booking online nowadays, so plan away and make it one to remember. Having time to research all the options is likely to result in cost savings as well as perhaps finding a more interesting location than you might settle for if you were in a rush, so take your time and find something great that will suit your new needs.

The World is a book, and those who do not travel read only a page.

Saint Augustine

99

Focus on your career

IT'S SURPRISING HOW OFTEN A new baby ends up meaning a new career for the mother. This may be in part due to old-fashioned workplaces not being very flexible towards new mothers, but perhaps also stems from new priorities and new ways of seeing the world. Certainly I've now come across a lot of women who radically altered their working life after having children: from changing their hours to setting up their own businesses. After my first child I went part-time but was happy to stay in my job. After my second child I was made redundant. I went for a new job but when I failed to get it I felt happy rather than disappointed and spent some time thinking about why that was. In the end I decided to change my life entirely and spend more time with my children while they are still small as well as pursuing my dream of writing for a living. So ask yourself: is your existing career still the right one for you or do you feel that the time has come to shake things up?

If you still love your job and want to do well at work then put aside a few of your breastfeeding sessions to keeping abreast of your industry – perhaps subscribe to a trade journal (or ask your workplace to pass on their copies when they've read them) or spend time on relevant sites so that you won't feel out of the loop when you go back to work. You can also run through some of the other suggestions listed here to make your re-entry to work impressive: from learning a new language to sporting a revamped wardrobe, having gained a relevant qualification or found some exciting new ideas on TED that you can implement at work. Your employer may even agree to pay for you to work on a valuable new skill while you are off work and be pleased with your commitment. Although if you are still on maternity don't let work *completely* take over – enjoy the break!

Choose a job you love, and you will never
have to work a day in your life.

Confucius

Get out!

100

Get out and about with
a breastfeeding sling

I've ERRED TOWARDS YOU BEING at home for most of these
suggestions, because a lot of the time you will be: nighttimes,
early mornings and evenings at the very least. Also, if you are out
and need to breastfeed, I am assuming you are probably doing
something fairly interesting anyway and don't need additional
ideas for things to do while you feed you baby. But there are
baby slings that allow you to breastfeed as you walk along and of
course this could free you up quite considerably: to go for walks,
to window-shop, to do most things in fact without needing to
stop when your baby needs feeding. I have tried it and I found
it a little tricky but it did work (plus I am a bit of a lazy person
and would rather sit down and relax while I breastfeed), so it's
worth you giving it a go. You may need to try out quite a few
models to get one that works for you, so you might want to find
a sling library or a good shop that can advise you on the best
model for your needs and shape as well as the age of your baby.
So when you're bored of being indoors and have used up all the
suggestions listed here: get out!

If you don't like the road you're walking,
start paving another one.

Dolly Parton

Resources

For breastfeeding and other parenting advice:
La Leche League: www.llli.org
Mumsnet: www.mumsnet.com
NCT (National Childbirth Trust): www.nct.org.uk

Other resources:
My website: www.melissaaddey.com
Funny, inspiring and important quotes: www.brainyquote.com
Writing a novel in one month: www.nanowrimo.org
Terrible first line of a novel award: www.bulwer-lytton.com
Inspirational talks: TED www.ted.com
The Guardian's bookclub: www.theguardian.
com/books/series/bookclub
Biological nurturing: www.biologicalnurturing.com

Your Free Book

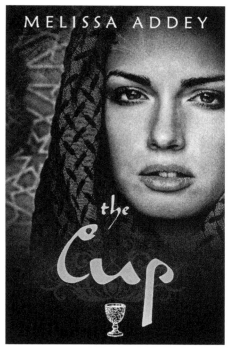

MELISSA ADDEY

the Cup

The city of Kairouan in Tunisia, 1020. Hela has powers too strong for a child – both to feel the pain of those around her and to heal them. But when she is given a mysterious cup by a slave woman, its powers overtake her life, forcing her into a vow she cannot hope to keep. So begins a quartet of historical novels set in Morocco as the Almoravid Dynasty sweeps across Northern Africa and Spain, creating a Muslim Empire that endured for generations.

Download your free copy at
www.melissaaddey.com

Thank you

THANK YOU FOR BUYING THIS book! I hope that some of the suggestions are useful to you and that they make your breastfeeding days more enjoyable. You can visit my Pinterest page and see the board for this book if you'd like to see some great pictures of mums breastfeeding while doing far more extraordinary things than I dared to suggest! www.pinterest.com/melissaaddey

If you liked this book and have a moment to spare (while breastfeeding, no doubt!) then I would really appreciate a review on the site where you bought it. Thank you for your help.

If you want to contact me directly you can email me at melissa@melissaaddey.com. I'd love to hear from you. Also remember to sign up for my mailing list and I'll email you that PDF of *10 things to do while Nappy Changing!* www.melissaaddey.com/nappies

Biography

I MAINLY WRITE HISTORICAL FICTION, AND am currently writing two series set in very different eras: China in the 1700s and Morocco/Spain in the 1000s. You can download a novella for free on my website: www.MelissaAddey.com

I worked in business for fifteen years before becoming a fulltime writer, during which time I developed new products and packaging for a major supermarket and mentored over 500 entrepreneurs for a government grant-making innovation programme. In 2016 I was made the Leverhulme Trust Writer in Residence at the British Library, which included writing two books, *Merchandise for Authors* and *The Storytelling Entrepreneur*. You can read more about my non-fiction books on my website.

I am currently studying for a PhD in Creative Writing at the University of Surrey.

I love using my writing to interact with people and run regular workshops at the British Library as well as coaching other writers on a one-to-one basis.

I live in London with my husband and two children.

For more information, visit my website www.melissaaddey.com

Current and forthcoming books include:

Historical Fiction
China
The Consorts
The Fragrant Concubine
The Garden of Perfect Brightness
The Cold Palace

Morocco
The Cup
A String of Silver Beads
None Such as She
Do Not Awaken Love

Picture Books for Children
Kameko and the Monkey-King

Non-Fiction
The Storytelling Entrepreneur
Merchandise for Authors
The Happy Commuter
100 Things to Do while Breastfeeding

Melissa Addey